Patterns in Education:
The Unfolding of Nursing

National Conference on Nursing Education

Pub. No. 15-1974

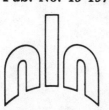

National League for Nursing

ISBN 0-88737-140-X

The views expressed in this publication represent
the views of the authors and do not necessarily
reflect the official views of the National League
for Nursing.

The papers in this volume were presented at the
National League for Nursing's First National
Conference on Nursing Education, "Patterns in
Education: The Unfolding of Nursing,"
Philadelphia, Pennsylvania, December 2–5, 1984.

CONTENTS

Patterns of Nursing Education

Perspectives on the Patterns of Nursing Education............3
  M. Louise Fitzpatrick

Nursing Education: Preparing for the Future...............11
  Martha E. Rogers

The Clinical Learning Experience: The Evolution
of the Nursing Work Force...........................15
  Mary Sue Infante

Mission for the Future of Nursing Education..............27
  Rhetaugh G. Dumas

Single-Purpose Institutions: Pro and Con

Can Single-Purpose Institutions Provide Baccalaureate
Education?...41
  Linda K. Amos

A Case for the Single-Purpose Degree-Granting College
of Nursing..49
  Sharon E. Bolin

A Disease Called 'Egalitarianism': Single-Purpose
Institutions for Nursing.............................57
  Julia A. Lane

Assessing Single-Purpose Institutions through the
Accreditation Process...............................65
  Sharon L. Diaz

Building a Knowledge Base

Dialectics of Theory Development........................71
Patricia Moccia

Being Informed: Nursing Resources for the
Information Age..79
Virginia Henderson

The Impact of Computers on Nursing....................91
Susan J. Grobe

State-of-the-Art Technology: Computers and
Curriculum 101
Gary D. Hales

Assuring Quality in Nursing Education

Strategies for Recruiting Graduate Faculty in Nursing
Service Administration................................119
Joan O'Leary

Credentialing: The Thread Between Licensure,
Accreditation, and Certification......................127
Robert V. Piemonte

New Opportunities in Nursing

The Corporate Connection: Multihospital Systems
Rekindle Commitment..................................143
Connie Curran

Marketing Continuing Education Programs in a Climate
of Cost Containment..................................153
Lawrence Litwack

International Nursing Education.......................163
Sister Rosemary Donley and Sister Mary Jean Flaherty

Preparing Clinical Specialists for Prospective
Payment..171
Lucille A. Joel

Patterns of
Nursing Education

PERSPECTIVES ON THE PATTERNS OF NURSING EDUCATION

M. LOUISE FITZPATRICK, EdD, RN, FAAN
Dean and Professor, College of Nursing
Villanova University
Villanova, Pennsylvania

As a contemporary nurse educator and a student of our history, I believe that nurse educators must provide leadership and direction to the field in designing and deciding what patterns of nursing education are sound, appropriate, and relevant for the future. This is an important part of our educational mission, and to abdicate to any other group within or outside of nursing is to be derelict in our responsibilities. As a consequence of the emphasis we have placed on clinical practice during the last 15 years, the role of the educator as the transmitter of knowledge, the developer of curricula, and, consequently, gatekeeper of the profession has taken a bit of a back seat. I call for today's educational leaders in nursing to stand up and be counted—and to attempt to pull into some coherent and relevant whole the fragmented system that continues to characterize preparation for nursing in this country. And I call on graduate programs to recognize the importance of preparing nurse educators in the knowledge and skills of education as well as in their essential subject matter—which is nursing.

Recently, I have been struck by the realization that nurse educators today seem to be less coversant with principles of teaching and learning as well as with the trends and the whole milieu of higher education in which nursing education resides. Despite the fact that we have a larger number of doctorally prepared faculty than ever before, they know less and less about higher education, curriculum development, and the educational process. This is a very real concern and an urgent matter.

The importance of charting our future course intelligently cannot be emphasized enough. To do this, a knowledge of our past and an understanding of the present are essential and useful. The major issues

3

confronting nursing education today have their roots in history and are the products of past decisions. Likewise, the ideas of many of today's nursing leaders are not necessarily new but have their genesis in another and earlier stage of our development. All that we are and have is inherited. Change is the only constant in our evolution.

PATTERNS OF THE PAST

The patchwork quilt that is American nursing education reflects our past responses to social, economic, and political forces that have acted upon us. The result have been both positive and negative. In many ways we have advanced the field far beyond our hopes and expectations. Yet, there continues to be a tendency for nursing education to revert to old and less relevant forms within this era of progress and change. As new patterns of nursing education emerge, many old forms hang on and drag the system downward. Sometimes they reappear disguised as new models of education, receiving acclaim and attention by those who are ignorant of the past and the regressive possibilities that these models carry with them. Other problems occur when we totally disregard the past and eliminate that which is sound and useful from older endeavors. Everything worth having—every goal worth achieving in nursing education—has been a struggle. The position of nursing education within the system of American higher education is the best example of a goal that was worth the struggle and that cannot and should not be disturbed or underminded as we move along.

We can point to results of our past efforts to advance nursing practice, education, and research. Examples are the quality of studies being conducted and the increased leadership that nurses are exerting on health care planning and policy development and through nursing's efforts in reaching well beyond the limits of our own organizations to influence health care in many arenas. We can also point to our achievements in developing the theoretical basis of nursing practice and expanding the body of knowledge that is unequivocally nursing.

But what of nursing education? We need a concerted effort to inform our educational decisions more fully, and we need to reacquaint ourselves with educational principles, values, and agenda that have always given nursing education its social and ethical significance. The only thing we cannot do is go backward and repeat the past. Today, we are confronted with important educational challenges and choices. We have moved out of the era when experimentation and proliferation of new programs and varied patterns of education can go unchecked. In an economy that limits the employment market for nurses, but also places more sophisticated requirements on the pool of individuals who will meet the health care needs of people in hospital, long-term, and community settings, we must rediscover, reinforce, and reaffirm our beliefs about nursing education and the essential elements of educational planning. Too many of these have been sacrificed in our bandwagon efforts to respond to every disenchanted group, every educational fad, every social and political influence, and every economic trend with yet another form of nursing education.

CONSENSUS ON CURRICULUM

There is no doubt that we must find ways, as quickly as possible, to "regularize" nursing education curricula without losing creativity in our programs or violating the freedom of schools and their faculties to meet objectives and develop competencies in their students in their own way.

Educational leadership in nursing is an imperative. We must get consensus on some essential points regarding curricula in schools of nursing so that our effort to make entry into professional nursing at the BSN level becomes a reality and a universal. This goal should not be thwarted through our own inattention to the curriculum question.

It is also important for us to keep in mind that if competencies, roles, and expectations of AD and BSN graduates are different, curricula must clearly reflect the difference and be appropriate to the respective levels. Ultimately, of course, the utilization of the AD and BSN graduates in the health care system is the single most important differentiating factor. The continuing dialogue and involvement of nurse educators and nursing service administrators in discussing curriculum matters has produced valuable results, and it must continue. A major dilemma is related to what the preferred construct for a sound professional nursing program should be at the level of the first professional degree. Some people assume that any program that awards a BSN and can get approval to operate is okay and on its way to accreditation.

Let me review some of our educational problems. Increasingly, the demands on baccalaureate education include attention to technological advance, but we should not sacrifice the important components of general and liberal education that undergird all professional curricula and which become increasingly important in the preparation of nurses. Despite a balance struck between classroom and clinical education, four academic years is becoming a more and more difficult time frame within which to prepare these students for the practice of the future. Even when the education is process oriented and the structure of the discipline is addressed rather than minute details of specific content, there is just not enough time.

Although we should not limit our imagination or our freedom to reconceptualize the field or limit our ideas and explorations, we must come to some decisions about what models of nursing education are appropriate for the future. In addition, we must challenge and curb the manipulation of nursing education by those who would have us lose our foothold in higher education by developing bastardized forms of preparation. Although we carry in our tradition a history of reform, we must guard against unsound change.

Fifty years ago, the model or ideal construct for curriculum and, therefore, the regularization of curriculum, was not a great problem. The National League for Nursing Education's *Standard Curriculum Guides* of 1917, 1927, and 1937 provided guidelines for uniformity of pattern, content, and time spent within a nursing program. And, of course, about 90 percent of the schools were then diploma schools.

Today, although we have American Nurses' Association standards for nursing education and National League for Nursing accreditation criteria, we have no real curriculum guidelines that help us to assure some consistency across programs. Consider the many routes to the professional degree, and the problems become obvious. We have four-year generic programs, upper-division generic programs, upper-division transfer programs, RN completion programs, two-plus-two models, generic master's and generic doctoral programs, external degrees, and a variety of patterns within so-called independent, single-purpose schools of nursing.

There is clearly more freedom and innovation in curriculum today, and much good has come from these decades of opportunty to develop professional nursing programs as we see fit. But there is also such difference in design that, as a practical matter, a baccalaureate student in nursing has an impossible time transferring into a similar program in another university once she or he has begun courses in the nursing major. I am not suggesting a new "cookbook" for curriculum development that destroys the valuable results we have achieved. But we must be able to provide evidence and assurance that there is some conformity among programs leading to the first professional degree. There is richness in diversity, but can we comfortably say that the objectives and content of the programs that provide the foundation for graduate study in any way resemble one another and are consistent?

I raise the curriculum issue repeatedly because I see it as central and as a prerequisite to setting our agenda for entry into practice in motion. It is a national concern and has not been attended to adequately for too many years. Our preoccupation with RN completion programs was necessary, but while we were trying to respond to the "RN question" in nursing education, we did not focus enough energy on the basic curriculum and what it should be. As a result, four-year programs as we have known them may be in great jeopardy. Let us not permit the curriculum issue to frustrate or limit our thinking, but let us not ignore it. It is crucial to our plan of action.

Baccalaureate education as the entry level for professional nursing practice is still debated in some parts of the country, but in most states it is no longer an issue. A growing number of jurisdictions have no hospital schools, and we can anticipate with some certainty that diploma education will soon take its rightful place in nursing's history. Simultaneously, we see the emergence of the hospital school in a new form—a single-purpose independent school of nursing that seeks to award a baccalaureate degree in nursing. Can or should this be tolerated? Can it be given positive sanction? Is it truly university education as we have come to define it? We must decide and do so quickly, for such mutations of the diploma school model are moving toward accreditation and calling themselves collegiate.

We know from our history that we can never get or expect complete agreement on all the questions and educational issues before us, but we *must* have consensus on major points and we should not violate basic tenets of education in the name of innovation.

QUESTIONS FOR THE FUTURE

I pose the following questions to be transposed into agenda items for nursing education for the future. What are the valid models of nursing education? Which have been created to serve a special purpose or group need and should be time limited and phased out? On what foundations are various models of nontraditional education developed? Which have relevance and staying power? Which are entrepreneurial efforts that exploit nurses and violate educational principles?

Within what kinds of higher education systems should nursing education exist—in liberal arts colleges, in universities without health centers, or only in academic health centers? Do we still need two levels of nursing? Do we have too many associate degree programs at a time when the employment market will exclude all but the best prepared at the higher levels?

If we continue to support two levels of nursing education—differentiating the roles of the professional nurse and the other, as yet unnamed category—can we also support two separate licensing mechanisms and cease our attempts to articulate the two kinds of programs? Or is greater articulation the answer?

Given the complexity of society, limited resources, and the requirements of nursing practice within a technological age, given a declining potential pool of students, how many basic and advanced nursing programs can we support? How many and what kind do we need? How can we prepare students for more home care and less hospital employment in a cost-effective manner?

At what point is educational diversity important, and at what points must we insist on conformity?

Since most nursing education programs do not exist within academic health centers, what collaborative models can be developed to provide for mutual support of practice and education without compromising the specific objectives of each?

Can we agree that the processes of education—teaching and learning—are as important as the content of our programs? If so, how do we reflect this in graduate programs that purport to prepare teachers of nursing, without diluting emphasis on clinical practice, research, and theory?

How can we ensure the liberal education of the student in a climate of high technology?

What checks and balances can be applied to the proliferation of doctoral programs that have neither the resources nor the prepared faculty to operate quality programs and do not go through an accreditation process?

What is the proper role of the National Council of State Boards of Nursing in influencing nursing education? How can we attenuate the agenda of that body to define practice, standards—and, soon, education for all of us—without the requirement that they either involve us or be held accountable to the rest of nursing and particularly nursing education? Are we willing to control our own destiny, or are we content to sit by passively and let others act upon us?

OPPORTUNITIES AND CHALLENGES

In order to answer these questions, we must be willing to openly discuss our differences as well as our points of agreement. This is dangerous, because so many "sacred cows" abound in nursing education, which are related to the problem of multiple entry routes into practice. We must be able to disagree without self-destructing.

These "sacred cows" are also some of our most popular buzz words: "career mobility," "career ladder," "educational mobility," and "curriculum flexibility." Too often, these are not adequately defined and are used inappropriately and interchangeably. We have confused these concepts for far too long. What we need is clarity about what we mean and what we believe and some consensus about how these beliefs are best expressed through curriculum patterns.

A priority for nursing education is to try to regularize—not necessarily standardize—curricula at specific levels without violating freedom, creativity, and educational opportunity. We need to clearly separate egalitarian and political motives, commendable as they may be, from the educational principles on which programs and curricula are established. Of course, our opportunities and challenges also carry risks.

Moving from an era of plenty to one of more limited resources creates its own adjustment problems. Nevertheless, it should give us impetus in deciding which of the many models of nursing education can and should survive.

Some positive factors may also be identified in an era of austerity. Retrenchment does not mean the cessation of development. There is precedent for using such time for productive reassessment, charting of future directions, and refinement of the products developed during periods of heavy external funding and rapid growth. Resetting our priorities will be the logical first step. In the past, economic stringency has helped to check the proliferation of substandard educational programs and has frequently yielded results in the application of standards and a view to quality as well as cost. Periods of retrenchment can also help us incubate new ideas. The important point is not to allow regression to the mean. Retrenchment can help us to understand that soft dollars should only be used for experimentation and the testing of models of education for the future—not to subsidize day-to-day operations. These are positives that emerge despite a conservative political climate, less money, and less students seeking careers in nursing.

The issues identified here are priorities requiring immediate attention from all of us and especially from our nursing organizations, for they are our collective power. We have no time for turf battles between ANA, AACN, NLN, or any other groups. We must identify the educational and curriculum leaders among us and demand their time and expertise in bringing us out of this mire. In the recent past we have sometimes denigrated curriculum and educational experts, while promoting the researchers, theorists, and clinicians. I am convinced that it is time for our educational leaders to again have their day in the sun. We need them desperately.

I was struck by the recommendations on the future direction of medical education made by the Panel on the General Professional Education of the Physician and College Preparation for Medicine of the Association of American Medical Colleges, chaired by President Steven Muller of Johns Hopkins University.[1] Among them are support for a more general education base in medical curricula; more integration of the humanities; and more attention to the development of skills of critical thinking and judgment formation. In short, the report calls for a radical shift—a revolution in traditional medical education. Likewise, the recent report that emerged from the special National Institute of Education Study Group on the Conditions of Excellence in American Higher Education, which considered the significance of the role of the humanities in higher education, points to the ongoing importance of preparing educated people as well as people prepared for a career.[2]

In nursing education, we have prided ourselves on our commitment to the values enunciated in both of these reports. Most nursing educators would declare that we teach critical thinking and that we integrate knowledge and skills. We would state that we base our professional curri-

---

[1] "Medical Schools Urged to Stress Critical Thought," *Chronical of Higher Education*, September 26, 1984, pp. 1, 15.

[2] U.S. Colleges Not Realizing Their Full Potential, Panel Says; Urges a National Debate on Quality," and Study Group on the Conditions of Excellence in American Higher Education, "Involvement in Learning: Realizing the Potential of American Higher Education," *Chronical of Higher Education*, October 24, 1984, pp. 1 and 35–49.

cula on a general education that includes a significant amount of liberal arts content. We in baccalaureate education have typically embraced the values of higher education in this country, and in many ways we are farther ahead than other fields.

But the tendency and temptation to slide back is greatly in evidence. Many curricula are giving less attention to all but those courses that directly support the nursing major. Some schools offering a BSN are not even based in colleges and universitites, but only purchase courses from them. If this isn't ignorance of our history and a backward step, what is?

If one agrees that nursing is a scholarly academic and practice field, one must also acknowledge that the placement of nursing education within the American college and university as an integral part of that social institution is the single most important historical and contemporary factor that we can identify as a reason for our progress as a profession. Universities exist to transmit extant knowledge and to inquire, debate, and generate theories that can be subjected to questioning and research. We must jealously guard the position we have earned in the American system of higher education and not be persuaded by zealots or faddists among us to give up what we have gained over the years in the name of flexibility, progress, or innovation.

NURSING EDUCATION: PREPARING FOR THE FUTURE

MARTHA E. ROGERS, ScD, RN, FAAN
Professor Emerita, New York University
New York, New York

A bit of ancient history seems appropriate to initiate these comments. Surely, all nurses were introduced to Hygieia and those other famous goddesses of health as early symbols of nursing. However, history reveals a somewhat different story than ones you may have heard or read. As a matter of record, Hygieia was a distinct personality by 600 BC (or perhaps earlier).[1] At least 200 years before Asklepios was introduced, Hygieia was a powerful and independent goddess responsible for maintenance of health. Her primary symbols were a serpent and an open hand. When Asklepios finally appeared he was only a hero, and heroes were not very important in ancient Greece. His function was to serve Hygieia and to do her bidding. He was very dependent on Hygieia, rarely appearing without her. Eventually (approximately another 200 years later), Greek males sought to overcome female dominance. Asklepios was promoted to a god and in time took the serpent for himself.

Masculine dominance continued in the Western world. In 1888, for example, Friedrich Nietzche stated that "when a woman becomes a

---

[1] See Marie-Therese Connell, "Feminine Consciousness and the Nature of Nursing Practice: A Historical Perspective," *Topics in Clinical Nursing* (October 1983), pp. 5-7.

scholar there is usually something wrong with her sexual organs.'' Nor has chauvinism ended yet. A recent article in the *New York Times Magazine* noted that ''interns do a lot of what they refer to as scutwork. 'Interns become great nurses,' as a surgery intern said.''[2] Then why haven't they been sued for practicing nursing without a license? Florence Nightingale's comment that ''medicine and nursing should not be mixed up; it spoils both'' needs to be remembered.

ENTRY LEVELS AND LICENSURE

Despite studies carried out ad infinitum and almost continuously throughout the present century, there has been very limited progress in support of an educationally sound and socially motivated system of higher education in nursing commensurate with changing times and human needs. The most significant change has been replacement of hospital schools with associate degree nursing programs. Concomitantly, valid baccalaureate degree education in nursing goes unlicensed and is only minimally differentiated from the associate degree and hospital-school level of preparation. The field of nursing has long had three entry levels to practice, and licenses for only two of these levels: the practical nurse level and the registered nurse level, for which associate degree and hospital schools prepare. Nursing has never licensed for the baccalaureate level, although the baccalaureate level is the cornerstone of nursing's educational system.

The myth that because all graduates of hospital schools, associate degree programs, and baccalaureate degree programs take the same licensing exam, they are therefore the same, approaches the ridiculous. With such logic one might properly ask why MDs and physician's assistants are not licensed according to one examination, or dentists and dental hygienists, or engineers and engineering technicians, and so on. Licensure exists to safeguard the public. There is critical need for the addition of a new license for the baccalaureate level of practice. Public safety requires it and professional credibility with other learned professions demands it. A grandfather clause for this new license must be limited to persons holding a baccalaureate degree with an upper-division major in nursing approved at the time of the student's graduation.

 An excellent baccalaureate nursing graduate is not the same thing as an excellent associate degree or hospital school graduate. In both instances excellence is determined by different criteria. Both groups should be equally excellent, but excellence will be manifest in different ways according to the nature and amount of knowledge each possess.

---

[2] Michael Harwood, ''The Ordeal: Life as a Medical Resident,'' *New York Times Magazine,* June 3, 1984. p. 46.

PROFESSIONAL EDUCATION

Nursing's survival as a knowledgeable endeavor demands that the education of nurses be squarely within educational institutions. Valid baccalaureate education requires a strong liberal arts foundation, substantive theoretical knowledge in the science of nursing, and the opportunity for students to demonstrate their ability to use their knowledge safely and effectively in service to people. Multiple community resources provide a range of laboratory settings. I agree with the recent report of the National Institute of Education, which recommended extending undergraduate programs beyond the usual four years in most professional fields.[3] I believe that the first undergraduate professional degree in nursing requires five years.

Regarding the evolution of professional education in nursing, I would add some words of warning. Hospitals are not educational institutions. They are but one of many resources for laboratory study in nursing and are highly inadequate settings for the broad scope of nursing. Moreover, it seems likely that in the future a decreasing percentage of baccalaureate and higher degree graduates will be working in hospitals. To those who would reinvent the wheel—beware! The historical accident that put nursing preparation in hospitals and outside the educational mainstream has been unfortunate for both nurses and the public.

It is imperative that we provide a valid baccalaureate education in nursing along with the degree. We must remember that our responsibility is to all people and is by no means limited to diminishing numbers of those hospitalized. Anti-educationism and dependency are untenable positions. Nursing is a learned profession—peer of other learned professions—unique in the phenomenon of its concern and in its substantive theoretical base.

Professional education in nursing is more than a piece of paper—it is located in and controlled by an institution of higher learning that includes a college of the liberal arts and sciences. It requires five academic years that include lower- and upper-division general education. The transmission of a substantive theoretical base in nursing science primarily at the upper-division level, with appropriate laboratory study in the art of nursing, gives identity to the student's major. And I would note that study in the physical, biological, and social sciences does not constitute study in the science of nursing. Rather, the liberal arts and sciences are requisites for all college students who seek to become educated people.

A qualified faculty prepared at the graduate level *in nursing* is essential if there is to be professional education in nursing. The possession of and the ability to transmit theoretical knowledge in nursing is indispensible. How one uses knowledge depends on the knowledge one possesses.

---

[3] Ezra Bowen, "Bringing Colleges Under Fire," *Time*, October 29, 1984. p. 78.

Functions are not nursing; they are how one uses nursing.

In these days of emphasis on cost containment, excessive charges by medicine and hospitals, budgetary battles, and the like, the public is properly concerned. Nurses are responsible for cleaning up their own act in terms of a society that both needs and wants knowledgeable nursing services.

Nursing's professionally educated population must be committed to people. They must be risk takers. They must be characterized by a mutual respect for differences. They must be imaginative and creative, and above all, they need a good sense of humor.

EDUCATION FOR THE FUTURE

High technology is having a large impact on nursing, as it is on the other areas of life. Automation, robots, the information revolution, and like events are not going away. Chatter of "high tech versus high touch" is fallacious. Both are meaningful adjuncts of practice in today's world. They are tools of practice. In the long term, if we educate for the future more jobs will be created than are destroyed. But for those who would maintain the status quo, the future is dim.

Before the end of this century, nurses can expect to be working in moon villages and space towns. Inclusion of "extraterrestrial" matters is a "must" in today's curriculum. Approximately 40 percent of RNs do not work in hospitals, and the percentage can be expected to increase in the future, particularly for baccalaureate and higher degree graduates in nursing. As Fritjof Capra has written, "we are trying to apply concepts of an outdated world view to a reality that can no longer be understood in term of those concepts.[4]

Autonomous nursing centers, independent nursing practice, nurse midwifery, birthing centers, outer space employment are emerging—and all without the fallacy of so-called medical backup. Only nurses qualified by baccalaureate and higher degree preparation in nursing are competent to provide the knowledgeable judgments necessary to public safety and to give appropriate direction to nursing's members with associate degree, hospital school, and practical nurse credentials. The direction of change makes imperative nurses' move toward scientific identity and social responsibility. Whatever the future of nursing may be, it will be within the context of rapid change, diversity, new knowledge, and new horizons.

---

[4] Fritjof Capra, *The Turning Point* (New York: Simon & Schuster, 1982).

THE CLINICAL LEARNING EXPERIENCE: THE EVOLUTION OF THE NURSING WORK FORCE

MARY SUE INFANTE, EdD, RN
Professor, School of Nursing
University of Connecticut
Storrs, Connecticut

As a nurse educator for so many years, I am accustomed to the accusation of being unrealistic or ivory-towerish in my beliefs about what type of nurses are needed by society and, particularly, about how to prepare them in educational programs. But I delight in the situation that currently faces us. Society is desperately reaching out for the kind of nurses envisioned and even described by many educators over the past few decades: knowledgeable, skillful, interdependent, decisive, creative, career oriented, scholarly, sophisticated, ethical, respectful, respected, and able to control their own destiny.

Yet, the image of the nurse held by the average person in society has changed little, if at all. That image is one of the nurse as helper, with some knowledge but less than the physician, anti-intellectual, skillful in routine tasks, and employed by hospitals. The nurse is viewed as a worker rather than a professional in the community.

The work force in nursing needs to hold onto and display the behavior of the former image, not simply for the sake of the profession of nursing but, equally important, for the sake of the quality of nursing care so sorely needed in society today. And educators need to shape that behavior. Let us look at the reality of the current situation in nursing practice as it fits into the health care delivery system and what the role of nursing education might be in shaping the practitioner we all desire.

15

THE STATE OF NURSING

Nursing is both flourishing and declining in the 1980s; it is in a period of peak need and lowered demand. Real need exceeds current supply. Yet, current markets are beginning to act as if supply exceeded demand. Some professional nurses are seeking employment, while nursing care to clients is inadequate, inefficient, ineffective, and in many instances inaccessible. Although the health care situation throughout the world is ready to tap the fullest potential of the field of nursing, the profession is struggling with frustration, burnout, unemployment, shrinking applicants to its programs, and justification of its own existence.

Ridiculous? Incredible? Ironic? Impossible! The situation in nursing and nursing education is a dilemma that requires *nurse intervention*. It is not unlike other situations that nursing has faced in its history, but it is more intense, more critical than ever before due to the nature and demands of the fast-moving pace of contemporary society. Nurse educators, who are central in deciding the practice of nursing and the direction of its practitioners carry a weighty responsibility. In any field, it is the educators who are expected to "plot the course." Out of the dreams of today come the realities of tomorrow. It falls on nurse educators to assess the current state of the art of nursing and to determine where it must go in the fast approaching twenty-first century. And, of course, all of this must be accomplished with shrinking budgets!

Currently, nursing has both the opportunity and the responsibility to practice in an independent and increasingly interdependent role in health care. Clients entrusted to the care of nurses require knowledgeable, astute assessments, decision making, and creative application of both the intellectual and psychomotor skills of the nursing process. Curative and preventive research has resulted in more people surviving illness and accident as well as more people immune to disease that they might otherwise have encountered. More people require maintenance and rehabilitative care; more people are living longer and require support in their advancing years.[1] Even death and dying is prolonged. Consequently, more people require the sustenance of comfort and the guarantee of dignity throughout the process of dying. In general terms, the current state of the art of nursing is that it is desperately needed by society, to a greater extent than ever before. The role of the nurse is heavily invested in prevention, the promotion of health, and the maintenance and rehabilitation of those with chronic and long-term disorders. Acute care or crisis-oriented care is of shorter duration and is heavily dependent on medical interventions. The role of the nurse is extending more and more into the community.

Having stated this, I cannot be as forceful or self-assured about nurses' readiness or willingness to take on these challenges and change their image.

[1] C. Cox, "Frontiers of Nursing in the 21st Century: Lessons from the Past and Present for Future Directions in Nursing Education," *International Journal of Nursing Studies*, 19, No. 1 (1982), pp. 1–9.

Nor can I be so unrealistic as to expect society to turn to nurses for the appropriate services. The public generally lacks the image of the nurse that would suggest these services, cause them to seek these services, and provide remuneration for these services.

Some reasons for the bewildering conflict we find ourselves in can be traced historically in both nursing and nursing education. We have enjoyed the wisdom of outstanding nurse leaders in our history; they practiced in an independent fashion, they led with visionary style. At the same time, our history is largely characterized by a reactive rather than an active role in shaping our image. Since colonial times, nursing has developed in this country by taking cues from non-nurses in a male-dominated environment. Nursing education began in the submissive, task-oriented atmosphere of hospital-based schools of nursing. The Great Depression further implanted the roots of this system by offering room and board to students, faculty, and practitioners of nursing in return for their service.

The influence of World War II manifested itself in a shortage of nurses at home and abroad, which led to the development of shorter, LPN programs and more task-oriented, nonprofessional care. After the fifties, of course, there was some movement of nursing education into the mainstream of higher education. Even in 1970, however, there was another stifling influence in the form of at least some of the recommendations of the National Commission for the Study of Nursing and Nursing Education, which suggested the granting of degrees in nursing by hospitals.[2] This document is still quoted as rationale for such endeavors by hospitals today, 15 years later. Why were we not more strongly and obviously influenced by so many other reports on nursing education throughout the years, such as those of Brown and Bridgeman?[3]

Even today, the clinical laboratory, the heart of any professional program of study, is still used in essentially the same way in all types of programs of study in nursing. Also, most nurse educators, while altering curricula toward a theoretical base in an admirable fashion, continue to teach in the same traditional way in the clinical laboratory. They teach as they have been taught.

CHALLENGES TO NURSING IN THE 1980s

As we proceed into the latter part of this century and ready ourselves for the next, I believe that nursing has the resources and the market to realize its full potential. I perceive this situation as a challenge rather than a threat. Nurse educators alone carry the heavy responsibility for preparing the practitioners of nursing of tomorrow. The society that they will serve is increas-

---

[2] National Commission for the Study of Nursing and Nursing Education, *An Abstract for Action* (New York: McGraw-Hill Book Co., 1970).

[3] E. L. Brown, *Nursing for the Future* (New York: Russell Sage Foundation, 1948); and M. Bridgeman, *Collegiate Education for Nursing* (New York: Russell Sage Foundation, 1953).

ing in affluence, demands, and expectations. We can, we must, and we will meet the challenges. Succinctly stated, we must produce highly competent practitioners of nursing while maximizing increasingly scare resources. Assessment of the challenges is essential before strategy and action can be designed.

For the first time in our history we face decreases in nurse faculty positions. Schools and departments of nursing are no longer escaping the stark reality of shrinking budgets. They are no longer immune to the loss of positions that our colleagues in engineering, education, and even liberal arts faced in the 1970s. As we are denied the opportunity to fill positions that are vacated by retirement or resignation, teaching and committee responsibilities fall to the remaining faculty. Thus, as faculty positions decrease, teaching loads increase.

This situation also increases student-faculty ratios in laboratory courses. Will the quality of teaching decline? Or will there be a resolve to explore teaching strategies that are yet unexplored by nurse educators—strategies that permit higher student-faculty ratios without sacrificing students' learning?

Competition for students is a truly intriguing challenge. Being primarily women, nurses and nurse educators have experienced firsthand the pain and the consequences of being treated as less than equal to males. The consequences have appeared in the form of low status, poor image, male domination, poor economic rewards, and generally inadequate educational facilities.

As the feminist movement began to take hold, nurses were in the forefront as proponents of women's rights—and that is as it should be. But what has happened? The number of women in higher education is increasing. Women are seeking lifelong careers rather than jobs for short periods of time. They are bright, energetic, and hardworking. They are interested in making career commitments—but they expect adequate salary and a lifestyle commensurate with their investment. Such goals and expectations are leading women into fields other than the traditional ones of teaching and nursing. Women are making inroads into pharmacy, engineering, business, and the like. These are women who previously might have chosen nursing. This phenomenon, coupled with the lowered birthrate of the past twenty years and the slow growth in numbers of males in the field, means less people are available to choose nursing as a career.

For the first time, there is competition for students—at least for qualified students. The number of applicants to programs in nursing is likely to stabilize at best and possibly to decline. We must enter the business of recruitment with a different perspective than ever before. We must have something attractive to offer the career-minded adolescent or the mature person returning to school for a delayed education. To attract these people to nursing and to retain them, we need to offer them stimulating programs commensurate with their intellectual abilities, affluent life-styles, and expectations regarding learning activities. Routine laboratory activities will not do; task-oriented care will not do.

The 1980s will see the climax in expectations of scholarship on the part of the nurse educator. More stringent criteria for academic preparation and subsequent scholarly achievement have gradually been required of faculty in schools and departments of nursing. Research and publication are now of the essence for tenure and promotion; more and more they are criteria for appointment.

Interestingly enough, the demand for scholarly productivity is coming at a time when budgets are tight, the number of positions is shrinking, and teaching demands are increasing. On balance, the competition for faculty positions is intensifying. Only the most able will survive, but even the most able will have difficulty meeting the myriad demands on time and energy. Again, the teaching strategies advocated and discussed in the seventies are likely to be pressed into action in the eighties, for expedient if not for philosophical reasons.

Continued viability of nursing depends on the visibility and credibility of nurses. That is, to achieve full professional stature and to realize full professional potential, nursing during the remainder of this century must first develop high visibility as a quality service, indispensable to individuals and communities. In health-related problems, congressmen, legislators, lawyers, health planners, and others should turn as quickly to nurses for input as they do to "doctors." Also, to increase visibility nurses must be assertive, forward looking, and articulate—always on the scene, always active. Second, nursing must be consistently credible. Attitudes, behavior, and accomplishments that are less than professional damage credibility. Credibility demands consistent, knowledgeable, and skillful services in a manner appropriate to societal needs. To achieve visibility and credibility, any professional person, including nurses, requires an educational preparation that fosters individuality, creativity, and problem-solving abilities. The most successful professionals know how to work with other disciplines in a team approach. These abilities must be inculcated, fostered, and nourished throughout the educational programs of the discipline.

The services of nurses, no matter how high in quality, and no matter how sorely needed, will not be recognized unless nurses are influential in both the governmental and private sectors. Influence is needed to obtain adequate monetary resources in lean economic times. The scramble is on for scarce resources. To achieve its full potential in the work force, nursing needs more educational resources in the form of buildings, space, equipment, support services; nurses need reasonable schedules, nurse-client ratios, and research monies. Clients need access to nurses and third-party reimbursement to pay nurses for their services in hospitals, long-term facilities, the home, and hospices. Requesting "more" of anything today is costly and futile. Nurses must learn to compete for resources along with the more experienced in this art. Increased political awareness and activism in government and on campus are essential for survival. It is imperative that the process of nursing education provide for the development of intellectual skills and practice opportunities to engage in political maneuverings for funds to support its goals—meeting the needs of clients in the health care delivery system and the needs of nurses in practice.

MEETING THE CHALLENGE: THE CLINICAL LABORATORY

How might we meet the challenges inherent in producing this knowledgeable, skillful, and sophisticated practitioner? Specifically, as educators, how can we achieve the goals so aptly stated in our program objectives? How can we grow ourselves, both personally and professionally, while proceeding with some degree of effectiveness and efficiency?

Focusing on the use of the clinical laboratory for this discussion is both appropriate and timely. Many would probably agree that dealing with the challenges nursing faces is much easier in classroom settings than in clinical settings. Yet, the clinical or "real-world" settings are the heart of any professional program of study. Furthermore, the clinical laboratory has long been cited as the reason nursing education needs more financial and faculty resources than other disciplines. Such claims are now more cliche than fact, especially in view of the fact that the results have been less than successful. Administrators in higher education as well as society at large are no longer likely to accept that nursing faculty have lesser credentials, more time, and more money than other faculty. So, an exploration of other means to our ends is appropriate.

History of the Laboratory Setting

The word *laboratory* is derived from the Latin *laboratorium*, meaning *workshop*. *Laboratory* is used to denote any place, situation, or set of conditions conducive to experimentation, investigation, and observation. During the first six centuries AD, the laboratory was primarily a place to make drugs and potions. In the Middle Ages, laboratories were also devoted to astrology. Physical and chemical laboratories developed in Europe in the eighteenth century along with experimentation and recording of results of science experiments. Gradually, laboratories were utilized to train young and newly inducted members into the trades.

As the laboratory became a place for students to learn, the focus on experimentation and research continued. At the present time, two major purposes of the laboratory exist in education for the sciences and the professions: (1) Laboratories are centers for experimentation and research, and (2) both simulated and real laboratories serve as centers of learning for students. Although several other professions have maintained the experimental focus in the clinical laboratory, nursing education has relied on a prescriptive, supervised approach to teaching in the clinical laboratory. There has been little opportunity for experimentation.

College Laboratory

Although laboratory in nursing education is used synonymously with clinical laboratory, the college laboratory is a setting complete with its own teaching and learning strategies. It is growing in importance as an essential facet of the "nursing laboratory." In fact, the use of the college laboratory should precede the use of the clinical laboratory for each clinical laboratory objective. This ensures a knowledgeable, skillful learner in each situation. Each skill objective, then, presupposes acquisition of tested knowledge, demonstration of skill in the college laboratory, and readiness for transfer of learning to the real situation. Both student and teacher must determine level of accomplishment in the college laboratory and readiness to move to practice in the clinical laboratory.

The college laboratory needs to become an established part of the sequence of teaching and learning activities and take an important place in the development of skills and attitudes. For this to occur, optimal use of the time, space, and equipment is needed. In relation to time, students should be free to practice skills when they are motivated to do so and when their personal and professional schedules permit. Hence, the college laboratory should be open to students during a wide range of hours, both during the week and on weekends. Also, laboratory personnel in the form of graduate assistants or baccalaureate-prepared nurses in the community should be available to staff the laboratory, both to serve as resource persons to the students and to facilitate a retrieval system. Faculty members should be available at selected hours during the week to reinforce teaching, respond to questions, raise additional questions, and determine students' readiness to move to the clinical laboratory.

College laboratories should be designed to contain both the space and equipment for media presentations and for simulation. The media portion provides students with the opportunity to listen to and view the application of concepts explored in class and through readings. Either commercially produced or faculty-produced tapes and videos portray the performance of the skill to which the student aspires. The simulation portion of the laboratory allows students to practice the skills themselves. Such skills include both the intellectual and psychomotor skills of the nursing process. Simulation can be portrayed through models and specially equipped dolls (such as Resussci-Anne), or through live, staged simulation of clients. The latter strategy has proven highly useful in some areas of medical education; it has much untapped potential for nursing education. The computer is another piece of equipment that is slowly making its way into educational laboratories. Computer-assisted instruction is also gaining popularity in college laboratories. A terminal connection between a college laboratory and a clinical facility that would provide client data for selection of clinical activities for faculty and students would save endless hours of commuting to determine clinical assignments.

In short, the college laboratory provides a wide range of opportunities for teachers of nursing to teach and for students to learn away from the disturbances, rigors, and demands of the clinical settings. It is a chance to practice apart from pressure prior to performing in a real situation. I am not suggesting that time in the college laboratory be used in lieu of clinical laboratory time, but rather that an appropriate balance be struck between the two and that each be used for a specified purpose—that one lead to and complement the other.

Clinical Laboratory

As noted earlier, budgetary constraints are making it virtually impossible to defend low student-faculty ratios. Unfortunately, since nursing and nursing education have tended to be more reactive than proactive, societal pressures to be more efficient may cause ratios to begin or continue to rise. I am concerned, too, about what will happen if teaching strategies fail to change. For some years now, I have encouraged a shift toward higher ratios and continue to urge nurse faculty to think this process through, be ready for it, plan for it, and head off problems whenever possible.

Student-faculty ratios can be increased without decreasing the quality of care or safety of clients. What is needed to accomplish this is a rethinking of the purpose of a laboratory and the teaching strategies to be utilized in conjunction with it. A laboratory is a place to conduct experiments, to pursue investigations, to make observations, to pose questions and hypotheses, and ultimately to apply research findings.

Interestingly enough, with high student-faculty ratios and more independent learning, students may, in fact, be better able to accomplish program objectives related to professional judgment, critical thinking, creativity, and problem solving. To accomplish such objectives, the faculty member provides guidance instead of supervision at the student's elbow. Students learn not by having the faculty member tell them what to do, but by having the faculty member guide them to appropriate selection of problem-solving tasks, which leads to an independent approach to testing theories. In fact, the teacher does not need to be present at all times in the clinical setting. Rotations need to be abolished; competency of performance as opposed to mastery of skills needs to be clarified.[4]

As far as safety to clients is concerned, recall the proposed use of the college laboratory. A measure of competency is assured before the student enters the clinical lab. Faculty provide for safety through what the student knows, not through what the teacher does. Teachers could thereby be guiding learning in a wide number and range of settings with a large number of students. There is nothing magical about a 5:1 or 7:1 ratio. In fact, in some such situations I have observed, learning was absent except by chance, and creativity was actually stifled. In raising student-faculty ratios, the goal is

[4] M. S. Infante, *The Clinical Laboratory in Nursing Education* (New York: John Wiley & Sons, 1985).

to produce more learning through quality teaching prior to the clinical laboratory and high expectations of students during the clinical laboratory.

A recent study produced some unexpected findings that tend to support this thesis. The study correlated a number of variables, such as student-faculty ratios and faculty members' tenure, doctoral status, number of publications, and years of teaching experience with students' pass rates on state boards.[5] Surprisingly, a significant finding was that the smaller the number of faculty in a given program and the larger the student-faculty ratios, the higher the pass rate! Could it be that these faculty members found creative ways to deal with their smaller numbers?

Clinical teaching should also permit theory to guide practice. Our entire approach to "what is nursing practice" is undergoing scrutiny and "correction of course." In other words, it is not a question of basic change but of altering the approach to achieve maximum potential. This "correction" is to make use of teaching approaches or strategies in which transmission of factual information is kept to a minimum and maximum use is made of theory to guide practice.[6] Nursing is a field of applied science. Let the research findings of a number of scientific fields determine our approach to assessment, underlie our plans, guide our interventions, and suggest questions for evaluations. *Let theory guide practice* and *let practice generate theory.* Think about this in relation to health teaching, compliance, and stress management as well as numerous other areas of nursing practice.

Such theoretical explorations lead to a substantially different approach to clinical teaching; namely, that all of the clinical laboratory is an experiment. All clinical laboratory activities involve the manipulation of variables. All clinical laboratory activities generate hypotheses. This approach eliminates questions about how to teach the research strand!

Undergraduates use applied, tested theory to determine practice; graduate students contribute to an expanded theoretical base for nursing and generate new theory through their research. To the graduate student, all clinical activities are clinical research. The undergraduate learns what experts in the field already know; the graduate student contributes new knowledge and insights to the field.

All too often, time spent in the clinical laboratory is utilized neither for learning what the setting has to offer nor in giving service to clients. Too much of the student's time is spent in "stumbling through the system"; looking for equipment; discussing with the faculty member questions that at best suggest lack of prior learning for transfer to the situation at hand; mimicking performance of other nurses or the faculty member in order to comply with unstated expectations; or performing routine tasks. Time spent

[5] M.D. Zanecchia, "A Study of the Relationships of Nursing Faculty Attributes, Faculty Productivity, Student Attributes and Selected Student Outcomes," unpublished doctoral dissertation, University of Connecticut, Storrs, 1981.

[6] E. Adams, "Frontiers of Nursing in the 21st Century: Development of Models and Theories on the Concept of Nursing," *Journal of Advanced Nursing,* 8 (1983), pp. 41-45.

in the clinical laboratory is costly and precious to the institutions or agencies, the clients, and the students. Faculty need to provide specific objectives for each portion of time spent in the clinical laboratory and ensure that the activities are related to the objectives. The *quality* or the use of time in the laboratory needs to be periodically reassessed.

Coupled with that is a need to reassess the *quantity* of time spent there. There needs to be specific purposes for being in the clinical setting. Yet, I am not necessarily recommending reduction in numbers of hours of lab. Clinical laboratory hours have reached dangerously low numbers in baccalaureate and master's programs. The pendulum has swung from long "work hours" to too few hours to learn. The process of socialization into the role of nurse or master's prepared nurse is endangered by too little exposure to the practice setting and its practitioners. Perhaps we are nearing the point of moderation, the pendulum is about to narrow its swing, and reasonable time allotments to the clincial laboratory will be determined to meet course, level, and program objectives.

All these efforts should be aimed at developing competency. All require sequencing of learning activities and provision of continuity in expectations and faculty guidance. All require the use of varied settings, at varied hours, and on varied days as opportunities for learning may present themselves. And, more and more, the client with a need for maintenance and rehabilitation will be found in the community. Community settings need to be utilized to a greater extent. Rather than look for pediatric experiences in acute-care settings, why not acknowledge that we manage to keep most children well and focus on well-child care? Rather than focus so heavily on care of adults and the elderly in acute-care settings, why not deal with major problems of provision and financing of care for long-term maintenance in the home? And the adolescents with serious drug and alcohol problems are out there in their homes and schools. Clinical laboratory time can be utilized most successfully in dealing with the health problems that are present in society— everywhere that people are.

TRANSFORMING VISIONS TO REALITY

I have addressed the philosophical and theoretical needs to test various approaches to utilizing a wide variety of clinical settings in order to produce the desired practitioner of nursing. What remains is to suggest ways to augment faculty guidance in the clinical laboratory. Budgetary demands as well as evolving role issues, such as faculty practice time, force nurse faculty to use their own time more effectively and to free themselves for research and writing activities. It is understandable that we sometimes forget that we, alone, need not be all things to all students, for as nurses we were led to believe that we should be all things to our patients, as if it were possible. We need to retrain our thinking, to become facilitators, influence others, and capitalize on resource people. In fact, by so doing, we just might broaden and enhance the learning of our students.

One way to do that might be to utilize the pyramid model of teaching, whereby an expert teacher works with less-prepared team members. The student has access to all levels of teachers. Another way to do this is to utilize clinical preceptors in clinical settings to provide some clinical guidance for students.[7] What better way to strengthen the ties between nursing service and nursing education than to involve practitioners in teaching? Clinical appointments could be utilized. Teaching assistants can and should be utilized apart from student interactions, particularly for teaching-related responsibilities such as item analyses, administering tests, grading, ordering books, and preparation of handouts and media.

Educational research studies are needed to test the efficacy of such arrangements. They are novel to us; but other disciplines have successfully utilized combinations of these strategies with a fair amount of success.

ASSESSING OUTCOMES

No discussion of clinical laboratory instruction is complete without attention to clinical evaluation. Clinical evaluation is, of course, necessary to determine if stated goals have been achieved by the learner. The entire process of evaluation is complex. Also, it is well known that during the evaluation process, anxiety levels rise while creativity levels decline.

Basically, the nurse educator needs to accept that evaluation methods should be consistent with teaching strategies. For example, if the learner takes an active role in shaping clinical activities, then the learner should be provided an active role in assessing the outcomes of those activities. Both shoud be nonthreatening.

Evaluation criteria should be directly related to course objectives. Formative evaluation of practice should be nonjudgmental, providing hints and suggestions rather than negative criticism. Summative evaluation and grading is necessary, but it should be reserved until the end of the course of study. There should be sufficient time to freely learn to explore without the constraints of being evaluated and graded. As for grading, most experienced teachers know well its unique set of problems. According to Dressel and Nelson, "There is no solution to the grading problem satisfactory to all concerned. Students would like all As, administrators would like few Fs, and the teachers would like to be left alone."[8]

SUMMARY

Professions will always be faced with the dilemma of how to provide quality programs while keeping costs down; of turning out practitioners competent

---

[7] M. R. Helmuth and T. D. Guberski, "Preparation for Preceptor Roles," *Nursing Outlook*, 28, No. 1 (1980), pp. 36–39.

[8] P. L. Dressel and C. H. Nelson, "Testing and Grading Policies, in *Evaluation in Higher Education*, ed. Dressel et al. (Boston: Houghton-Mifflin Co., 1961), p. 251.

to meet current and future needs while keeping tuition costs within reason; and of preparing for tomorrow's practice without losing sight of today's demands and resources. These points require continual reexamination. My plea is for openness and creativity of thought on the subject. We may possibly be able to accomplish our goals just as well through different means; and quite possibly we may be able to improve our achievement of goals through unique approaches. Let us not merely teach as we have been taught.

In moving programs of nursing to a college or university setting we not only changed our location or address, we supposedly changed our mission. We aspired to produce an educated person as well as a capable practitioner. Bartlett Giamatti, president of Yale University, reminds us of the purpose of higher education:

> While securing a cup of coffee with a reporter in a line at a cafeteria-style restaurant in New Haven recently, Mr. Giamatti explained his own view of Yale's mission in animated fashion: "Not to make one technically or professionally proficient, but to instill some sense of love of learning for its own sake, some capacity to analyze any issue as it comes along, the capacity to think clearly, regardless of what the subject matter must be." So transfixed was the woman behind the counter with this eruption that she poured almost the entire contents of a coffee pot into a single cup.[9]

In our own field as well, visionary leaders articulated educational goals for nurses. Florence Nightingale reminds us of the purpose of nursing education:

> For us who nurse, our nursing is a thing which, unless in it we are making progress every year, every month, every week, take my word for it, we are going back. The more experience we gain, the more progress we can make.... After all, all that our training can do for us is teach us how to train ourselves.[10]

Nurse educators must manipulate the clinical laboratory settings and its inherent opportunities to provide society with that type of practitioner of nursing.

[9] *New York Times Magazine*, March 20, 1983, p. 42.
[10] F. Nightingale, *Florence Nightingale to Her Nurses* (New York: Macmillan Co., 1914).

MISSION FOR THE FUTURE OF NURSING EDUCATION

RHETAUGH G. DUMAS, PhD, RN, FAAN
Dean and Professor, School of Nursing
University of Michigan
Ann Arbor, Michigan

Tremendous progress has occurred in nursing education. Nevertheless, some thorny problems have been accumulating over time, and others have recently begun to emerge. We have been challenged to give more attention to the identified problems—to move faster to eliminate them. We have also been cautioned not to repeat the problems of the past—that in our efforts to resolve current problems and issues, we not "reinvent the wheel."

PROGRESS AND PROBLEMS

By now there should be no doubt that nursing education is indeed unfolding. Over the past 20 years, its unfolding has been dramatic. It is said that nursing education has undergone a revolution since 1960.

We have succeeded in moving nursing education into institutions of higher learning. A goal that was pursued for over a century has been achieved in just the past two decades. In 1960, 83 percent of the new graduates were educated in hospital schools of nursing. By 1980, this trend was completely reversed: 83 percent of the new nursing graduates received their education in colleges and universities, and one in three practicing nurses had a baccalaureate degreee.[1] The number of master's

---

[1] J. C. Gornick and L. S. Lewin, *Assessment of the Organizational Locus of the Public Health Service Nursing Research Activities* (Washington, D.C.: Department of Health and Human Services, September 1984).

prepared nurses increased by over 300 percent in the nine years between 1964 and 1975, and the number of nurses enrolled in doctoral programs rose by 500 percent between 1960 and 1980. Although the absolute numbers are still inadequate to meet our current needs, we are nevertheless moving forward.

As nursing education has unfolded, nursing research has been rapidly coming of age, and we have witnessed important improvements in the standards for and quality of nursing practice, nursing education, and nursing research. Our leadership has been growing and exerting more influence in health care planning and policy decisions. We are reaching out beyond the boundaries of nursing programs to contribute and influence events in our colleges and universities, in our communities, states, and nation. Our influence is becoming visible in many other aspects of life in this society. This influence must be strengthened and expanded, but we have made a good start. Theoretical frameworks for practice are expanding, and we have begun to identify knowledge that is unequivocally nursing.

Whether we like it or not, we have an impressive review and evaluation process to monitor the quality of nursing education programs under the National League for Nursing accrediting body. The dramatic advances that we have witnessed over the past 20 years have been influenced by the improvements and expansion in baccalaureate education for nurses, by the initiation and development of the alliance between nursing and junior colleges that led to the rise of the associate degree programs, and by the decline of hospital-based nursing programs.

The federal government has played a critical role in the unfolding of nursing education over the past 20 years. The Nurse Training Act of 1964 was the first comprehensive federal legislation to provide funding resources for nurse training and nursing education. Over the years, the provisions of this legislation have been supplemented by provisions of the Public Health Service Act, which authorizes funding for research projects and research training fellowships. The Nurse Training Act of 1964 was expanded by amendments in 1968, 1971, 1975, and 1979. This legislation has expired, and our most recent efforts to obtain renewal legislation met with pocket veto by President Reagan shortly before the 1984 elections.

From the time of the passage of the Nurse Training Act to 1982, appropriation for nursing education and research programs totaled over $1.6 billion. The mid-1970s were the most liberal years. The level of funding has declined since that time, except for 1980 and 1983, when the appropriations for research were improved. Significant changes in federal health policy and program regulation have put this resource for nursing education at risk of even more dramatic cuts or complete phaseout.

This is part of the new federalism that intends to shift the financing for health professions education from the public to the private sector. In so doing, the government policymakers have taken the position that the current institutional capacity of health professions education is adequate to produce the needed supply, and that market forces will be sufficient to influence the production, specialization, and distribution of health professionals across the various professions.

Efforts intended to increase the funding support and put nursing research in the mainstream of scientific investigation within the federal sector also met defeat with the veto of the bill to reauthorize the National Institutes of Health and establish a National Institute of Nursing. Unless these trends are reversed, it is uncertain what federal support will be available for nursing education and nursing research in the future. This is occurring at the same time that we are faced with targeted budget reductions as part of the retrenchment programs in our colleges and universities and that the new prospective payment systems of reimbursement for Medicare are having a profound and pervasive impact on the structure and operations of hospitals and the entire health care system.

Although the future of nursing within the prospective payment system is not yet clear, there are clear indications that neither nursing service nor nursing education will be able to continue business as usual. We must attend to problems stemming from the variable patterns of nursing education (diploma, associate degree, and baccalaureate). The distinctions among them are unclear. They are not differentiated by licensure. Some have identified this as a problem of sufficient concern to warrant consideration of separate licensure for graduates of baccalaureate and higher degree programs.

A number of additional problems plague nursing education. Nursing education programs are mushrooming without an adequate supply of qualified faculty. Nurses who lack college degrees are teaching in some of our nursing education programs. Insufficient numbers of nurse faculty are prepared as educators, in the broadest sense—they may be well versed in the subject matter of nursing, but they lack the perspective of higher education. We need faculty members with credentials appropriate to their fields of instruction and more doctorates in nursing. There is a perceptible lack of consistency in the standards for and quality of nursing education programs. Among the faculty and students of these programs, concern has been expressed about the emergence of single-purpose organizations for the education of professional nurses. There are variable models among the single-purpose organizations; they are not all the same. The emergence of these programs is a perplexing problem that we have yet to resolve.

There are obviously other problems that I have omitted here, but these are enough to give an overview of the work that lies ahead. Having cited progress and some problems in nursing education, let me summarize some of the challenges that are implicit in them.

CHALLENGES TO NURSING EDUCATION

We are challenged to find more effective ways to deal with the issue of the multiple patterns of nursing education. We hear the dramatic statement that if forced to choose, we should go with the technical nurse— because of her ability to administer oxygen and carry out other vital technical procedures. The implication is that the technical nurse might do more for survival of patients than those whose nursing education has taken other paths. Of course, this statement has been appropriately challenged. The implicit anti-education theme is that what is really critical is the nurse's technical skills. This denies nursing as a learned profession.

The question of whether we can afford to continue all the varied patterns of nursing education no doubt elicits both positive and negative responses. But we are indeed challenged to at least continue the debate. Many are pushing for a definitive decision. But who decides and on what basis?

We are challenged to consider the full range of issues associated with the desire among some to have separate licensure to differentiate the pattens of nursing education. We are challenged to expand our perspectives; to think more about policy; to learn to distinguish between policy and politics; to see policy development as an approach for resolving some of the problems that confront us. We are challenged not to take things for granted—keeping in mind that there are no random happenings in the universe. We must seek to understand the nature of our problems, how they have come about, what the policy issues are. We must frame our arguments and activities so that they hit at points in policy. Policy relates to ideals, values, equity, community—all of which are vital parts of what we must deal with in effecting the changes that we are seeking today and for the future.

We need to focus more on what nurses think and how they think. We are challenged to broaden our perspective, to be more futuristic. Many of the problems that seem to loom so heavily on our horizons today may not even be relevant in the future!

For example, we are accustomed to thinking about nursing in hospitals, yet increasing numbers of nurses will work outside of hospitals in the future. Today 40 percent of the RNs are working outside hospitals, and this portion will undoubtedly increase over time. To expand our visions, to chart our own future course, means that we must reexamine our tradition. Older and less relevant forms must change. New patterns must not be undermined by outmoded approaches. Indeed, in times of broad, rapid change such as we are witnessing today, the most pressing challenge to us in nursing education is to ensure that our positive gains will not be eroded and that we will be capable of continuing progress in an increasingly competitive and cost-conscious environment. To meet this challenge, we must not ignore our problems, but neither can we afford to get bogged down in them. Most of our problems are a function of growing pains, and with committed, sustained, cooperative efforts, we can resolve many of them.

MISSION FOR THE FUTURE

We have the potential to meet effectively the challenges of today and those of the future. It is our professional duty to mobilize and fully exploit our inherent capabilities, to overcome our shortcomings, and to build on our strengths. That is at the core of our mission for the future of nursing education.

In endeavors to fulfill this mission, we must be careful not to lose perspective on the world in which we live and work. For, our relationship to that world—which provides the context for nursing education, nursing practice, nursing research, and all of our health-related activities—will ultimately be the major determinant of progress or lack of progress in the future.

In a time of rapid social and economic change, survival and progress will be proportionate to our capability to adapt to a world in transition. Barnet states that:

> Every generation is by definition an era of transition, but our own time portends bigger changes in the organization of the planet than we have had for at least 500 years. A crisis of values has swept across both capitalist and socialist worlds. The rapid process of decolonization following 400 years of imperial conquest in Asia, Africa, and Latin America is far from completed. Profound struggles are taking place or are in the offing—between rich and poor nations over their share of the world product, within the industrial world over sharing resources and markets, and between cities and regions within nations over access to food, fuel, minerals and water. The world is already in the midst of a transition to a post-petroleum civilization.[2]

In addressing the scarcity of natural resources, the author describes how circumstances surrounding the energy crisis have led to the global division of labor and the rise of multiproduct, multinational corporations that are having tremendous influence on the world economy. This is having very important implications for the lives of people all over the globe, and we in America are not excluded.

Megatrends is a frequently cited reference among nurses these days.[3] But what we have chosen to highlight is interesting. For example, the "high-tech/high-touch" cliche, if you will pardon the expression, is out

[2] Richard J. Barnet, *The Lean Years: Politics in the Age of Scarcity* (New York: Simon & Schuster, 1980), p. 19.

[3] John Naisbitt, *Megatrends: Ten New Directions Transforming Our Lives* (New York: Warner Books, 1982).

of character for this learned profession that professes to get *beneath* the skin of people through piercing intellectual explorations and rational analysis. The proposition that the congregation of people in shopping malls and on dance floors represents a need for "high touch," which is evoked by high technology, is not convincing. In my opinion, this touching business is a rather superficial issue.

Megatrends says a lot more than that, though. Perhaps it is the tendency to deny the realities of life in the world today that accounts for inattention to information which sheds greater light on the desperate economic and social problems that are forcing dramatic changes in our immediate environs. Understanding the nature of these changes that have already begun to affect our lives and that will inevitably force significant changes in nursing education is part of our mission for the future of nursing education.

Megatrends and several other treatises that address the social and economic trends in our society call to our attention the decline in our national economy, which is due to a significant degree to changes in the world's economy. Just a few years ago, the United States was the most dominant force on the world economic scene. Our national economy was isolated and essentially self-sufficient. It was fashionable then to worry about poverty amidst great affluence. Today, the United States has become part of an interdependent global economy, in which the economy of any one nation is influenced by the operations and markets of all others. We are no longer the dominant economic force, and we have lost our claim to the highest standard of living in the world.

Domestic policy and economic strategies designed to rebuild our national economy are having their repercussions in every aspect of American life. The gap between the haves and have-nots is widening as the federal government unloads the burden of social programs and deregulates services to the public, allowing market forces to control their availability and quality. The federal government has instituted prospective payment systems and diagnosis-related groups to control costs of hospital care for Medicare recipients.

From my perspective, some of the internal problems of the profession that we agnoize about so much pale in the face of the tremendous challenges imposed by the broad and rapid social, economic, and political changes that we must be prepared to manage. It has been said that we need to choose which pattern or patterns of nursing education should survive. Do we really? I think that there is a place and a need for associate degree programs as well as baccalaureate programs—the former defined as preparation for the technician, the latter as preparation for beginning *professional* practice.

Those of us who are committed to providing for this mix should put our efforts toward developing these patterns. We should leave to the proponents of the single-purpose nursing education organizations the responsibility of rationalizing that pattern in light of current and emerging trends, issues, needs, and standards for higher education in general and higher education in nursing specifically. We have provided them very clear and logical arguments about the pitfalls. Now it's up to them.

We should target our challenges regarding single-purpose institutions to the policy issues: What should be the patterns of nursing education for the future? What changes need to be made in existing patterns? What are to be considered necessary conditions? What conditions are sufficient to qualify as acceptable models? Why are these models necessary or sufficient? Where do single-purpose organizations fall short on such matters of policy?

Let me warn that we should not spend too much time on this issue. We must not lose sight of the fact that the mass of nursing education programs are in institutions of higher learning. They are *not* in single-purpose institutions. We must ultimately have enough flexibility to allow for deviance. Otherwise, many creative opportunities will be lost. For example, the disadvantages or advantages of the various patterns of nursing education are after all empirical questions. Let's put them to the test!

Success in fulfilling our mission for nursing education in the future will require the capability to manage change effectively and efficiently. Effectively means doing the right things; efficiently means doing what you are already doing better and at lower cost. Managing change effectively in this new era of stringent social and economic constraints means questioning whether we are doing the right things. This raises yet again fundamental questions about the nature of nursing and, accordingly, the nature of nursing education. It means getting down to basics. To aid in this process, let me remind you of the classic works of Virginia Henderson.[4]

Managing change effectively demands that we question the nature of our organizations for the education of nurses—their missions, goals, and the priorities for the allocation of scarce resources. It means reorientation to norms and cherished values, refocusing efforts, reevaluating our standards and systems for rewards. It means coming to grips with the realities that will prohibit us from doing all that is needed or that we desire to do.

Nurses have embarked on the age of scarcity, and we can no longer yield to the longings to be "angels of mercy"—all things to all people. We will be forced to make hard choices. Are we prepared to make them, and are we equipping the future generations of nurses to make them? What are we doing now and what must we do in the future to ensure informed rational choices? Let me suggest a few of the steps that occur to me.

---

[4] Virginia Henderson, *The Nature of Nursing: A Definition and Its Implications for Practice, Research, and Education* (New York: Macmillan, 1966); and Virginia Henderson and Gladys Nite, *Principles and Practice of Nursing* (New York: Macmillan, 1978).

Today, right now, we must ensure that faculty and students thoroughly understand the principles of the prospective payment system and all the implications that prospective payment and diagnosis-related groups have for nursing education—its principles and goals, the curriculum, teaching approaches, research. This system is only the tip of the iceberg. Similar strategies will surely continue to emerge for all parts of the health care systems. We are challenged to reexamine our existing programs and make the changes that are necessary to incorporate the theory and the practice approaches to enable nurses to function competently in the cost-conscious environment in which they will live and work.

Course offerings at all levels in the educational system should be reviewed and revised as necessary to enable our students to develop the commitment, the mentality, the knowledge, and the technical skills that are, or will be, necessary to balance the goals of competent, excellent, and caring service to humankind with those of efficiency and reduction of costs. This will be a challenge for years to come. We must include content that will inspire and enable our graduates to assume active roles in efforts to improve the quality of nursing care, of health care, and the quality of life in their organizations, communities, and nation and to share the diligent work needed to make this a better, healthier world in which to live.

We must see that our programs of study equip nurses to manage in a competent and ethical manner the dilemmas that will undoubtedly intensify under conditions of fierce competition for limited resources. They must be able to cope effectively in situations in which they may feel pressured to choose courses of action that fall short of their ideals.

We are challenged to prepare nurses who can organize and manage work and resources effectively and efficiently. This will be critical not only for those with clear intention to prepare for formal administrative roles, but for all nurses preparing for any role, for they must share responsibility and be accountable for high-quality performance. There is a critical need for programs to prepare nurse administrators with capabilities that will be required in the new economic era. We must gear our research to problems of practice in the era of the prospective payment system. This will be critical, for example, if we are to develop case mix profiles, determine the nursing requirements for the case mix, develop appropriate and cost-saving staffing patterns to meet the nursing requirements of the case mix, and develop schema for quality assurance that are correlated with length of stay and nursing cost.

We need more studies to identify and measure factors that affect the utilization and cost of nursing resources. In our schools and departments of nursing, we are challenged to work harder to become partners with our colleagues in schools of medicine and those in hospital administration and health planning. We must ensure that our contributions will be helpful in maintaining the financial viability and prominence of the academic medical center—a goal that both today and in the future poses the kinds of challenges that will require working together. Nursing can give our hospitals the cutting edge in the competitive market, so nursing educators are challenged to pair up with nursing service administrators to get the state of the art in nursing to the bedside.

There are a number of other challenges that we must prepare to meet. Hospital administrators, in efforts to control costs, will no doubt restrict or reduce staff to levels that can be specifically defended, based on well-measured outputs. In some cases this may mean reduction in the number of nurses by whatever means necessary. But it might also mean a reduction in the level of preparation and experience of nurses who are retained or hired. Unless it can be demonstrated that such actions are counterproductive to goals of patient care or that overall they are not cost saving, administrators may feel justified in cutting nursing costs by whatever means possible.

Our challenge will lie in enabling nursing to develop the kind of data base that will be needed to demonstrate the cost and value of nursing care and to assess the impact of educational preparation and experience on costs and quality. We must develop effective approaches for raising the level of political sophistication among nurses so that they can lobby for the goals and practices they deem necessary and negotiate for turf and resources to achieve them.

Reimbursement for nursing services is a critical issue with which we must deal. More narrowly defined boundaries for nursing practice are emerging. We are challenged to develop the strategies and the support to ensure that the progress we have made in developing professional nursing will not be eroded and to ensure that we can move forward with our colleagues in the health sciences, the hospital, and the rest of the university and compete favorably outside as well.

The school or department of nursing is challenged to identify opportunities that are provided by the changes in health care arenas. Cost-cutting initiatives need not limit opportunities for significant contributions from nursing through existing and expanded roles. In fact, new approaches and change might do much to raise job satisfaction and morale. The challenge to reexamine, redefine, and refocus our thinking can be progressive. To take advantage of new opportunities will mean taking an active rather than a reactive stance.

Whether it is realized now or not, hospitals are going to need better prepared nurses to assume the responsibilities that are demanded by prospective payment systems and the other economic strategies that are yet to come. Nurses can be a vital force in helping hospitals expand the scope of services beyond traditional inpatient and ambulatory services and at the same time offer exciting opportunities for faculty practice and clinical practicums for students in models for the vertical integration of health services.

We must begin now to question the necessary educational level for the beginning nurse. Our colleagues in nursing service are feeling insecure about the capability of new undergraduates to manage the intensity of work in the emerging environment. We need to question whether admission to our nursing schools should be postbaccalaureate rather than post-high school.

There will be new positions and opportunities in community settings and in entrepreneurial activities. It is said that market forces will influence the direction of health care, and market forces will influence the production and distribution of health professionals in the future. This is to rationalize the pullout of the federal government from responsibility for broad public programs to ensure the health and welfare of the citizens of this country.

A theoretical assumption in microeconomics is that under conditions of perfect competition, when numerous competitors are left unrestrained to win the favor of customers, two major criteria for an effective market will be optimized simultaneously: the customer will be best served, and the competitor will gain maximum profits or benefits. But we are told that perfect competition is seldom observable, and in most situations the two criteria are not optimized simultaneously. Many competitors seek their benefits through satisfying customers. But in many other cases, competitors seek their benefits through strategies to influence the customer to buy what they have to sell. Some may even withhold the truth or some part of the truth about that which they are selling.[5]

Furthermore, we all know that the market favors those who can afford to buy. We know what these changes in health care enterprises will mean for the economically deprived and socially disadvantaged people whose causes and needs we have traditionally advocated. Times of scarcity are invariably times of struggle. In contemplating our mission for the future, we must not neglect the responsibility to engage the struggle to make this a better world for nurses that we have or will educate and for the public that we all endeavor to serve.

The recommendations of the ultraconservative Heritage Foundation to President Reagan were recently reported.[6] The foundation members urged the president to launch a top priority battle against the comparable worth theory for achieving pay equity for women. They also recommended that the Justice Department require federal officials to submit for advance censorship their writings and speeches for life; and that the Justice Department work to end federal set-aside programs to ensure minority businesses access to government contracts. Their suggestions for Congress included persuading it to restore the death penalty for murder, treason, and espionage; eliminate the insanity defense in

[5] H. I. Ansoff, *Strategic Management* (New York: John Wiley & Sons, 1979), p. 15.

[6] Michael J. Sniffen, *Philadelphia Inquirer*, December 3, 1984.

criminal cases; limit federal voting rights enforcement to instances where there is discrimination against minority voters; end court-ordered busing; oppose a bill expanding the definition of housing discrimination; oppose the bill to extend civil rights guarantees to an entire state, local, or private facility if part of it receives federal aid; repeal laws against price fixing; and step up prosecution for pornography. If implemented, these recommendations would turn the clock back many years on our society, and the lives and careers of all nurses today and in the future would be negatively affected. Our mission in nursing education is to understand the nature and impact of such trends and marshal forces to reverse them.

Finally, in pursuing our mission for the future, we must not fail to address what Barnet calls the most serious energy crisis in the world: "The depletion of human energy that results from hunger and malnutrition—when the brain receives too few calories or too few proteins to think and the body too few to act. Damaged adults producing damaged children generation after generation."[7] We know that in times of scarcity the very old, the very young, minorities and women, and the mentally and physically handicapped suffer the burden of the economic hardships.

The Heritage Foundation is not concerned with such problems. But we are, and we must reflect these concerns in our agendas for the future. We are part of an admirable, socially significant, and highly relevant profession. We have come again to a critical juncture in our development, and the paths for the future cannot be selected randomly. We must organize for strong and sustained collaboration to chart our future course. I have faith in our capability, and I have great hope for the future.

---

[7] Barnet, *The Lean Years.*

Single-Purpose Institutions: Pro and Con

CAN SINGLE-PURPOSE INSTITUTIONS PROVIDE BACCALAUREATE EDUCATION?

LINDA K. AMOS, PhD, RN
Dean and Professor
University of Utah College of Nursing
Salt Lake City, Utah

The term "single-purpose institution" has been bandied about in the last year or so without any clarification of what these institutions are like. When it is analyzed, however, it becomes clear that it is an inappropriate description of the issues usually under discussion. The development of nontraditional baccalaureate programs in nursing in institutions that have a primary mission of providing clinical services to patients and also have a diploma program in nursing has created this controversy. Several program models have emerged or are under discussion. The characteristics of these programs vary significantly; yet they all have been clustered under the one descriptive phrase, "single-purpose institutions," when the term hardly characterizes any of them.[1] Changes in health care delivery, the need for a greater base of knowledge and skill in nursing, and the movement toward baccalaureate preparation as the minimal base for professional practice, along with major financial considerations, have motivated the development of these new programs. There is no doubt that there is need for change and that many institutions have to face the reality of some transition. The larger question is how to make

---

[1] Bernard F. Rodgers, Jr., "Educational Mobility for Hospital Schools of Nursing," paper presented at the American Hospital Association Conference, Chicago, Illinois, March 17–18, 1983.

the necessary changes while preserving the essential qualities of a baccalaureate degree program in the process.

I will first describe some of the models of baccalaureate education programs in nursing. Then I will focus on the elements of program development that raise major concerns. Finally, I will conclude with some general
statements about the essential elements of baccalaureate preparation for
professional nursing and why they are critical to the development and
maintenance of quality professional preparation for nursing.

MODELS OF BACCALAUREATE PROGRAMS

Stand-Alone Hospital Degree Program. A hospital with a diploma program in nursing obtains degree-granting status through state provisions
and offers a baccalaureate degree in nursing. Students are admitted after
completion of the liberal education or preprofessional base.

Joint Hospital/College Degree Program. A hospital with a diploma program contracts with a college in the community for a cooperative arrangement to offer a baccalaureate degree. The degree is awarded jointly,
and each institution seeks its own separate accreditation from the regional
accrediting body.

Degree/Diploma Completion Program. In this model, there is a contractual agreement between a college and one or more hospital diploma
programs for the offering of a baccalaureate degree in nursing. This
model leads to both a diploma and a BSN, both awarded by a college.
The hospital does not seek separate accreditation. An essential component
of this model is a detailed agreement on transfer of hospital school courses
into academic credit in the college.

Hospital Degree Program with a Cooperating College. In this model,
the hospital obtains degree-granting status and grants the degree alone.
The hospital has a contractual arrangement with a college for the liberal
education and preprofessional courses.

The common theme among all the models cited is related to the fact
that a hospital diploma program either sought its own degree-granting
status or connected with a college for the purpose of granting a baccalaureate degree. Many programs are currently developing in each of
the categories described. The change has been fairly rapid, and questions
abound in professional circles about the validity and quality of such programs. Have these programs merely taken a diploma program and added
some liberal arts courses? Has the nursing curriculum changed sufficiently
to reflect the essentials of baccalaureate education? How can a hospital,
whose primary mission is patient care services, also become an educational institution and protect all the values of higher education, when

the potential for conflict in priorities is so great? Is it appropriate and ethical to utilize dollars spent for patient care to subsidize nursing programs of this nature? How can a hospital provide the type of environment found in colleges and universities, including the presence of libraries with literature from all branches of knowledge, centers of various sorts, and broad opportunities for pursuit of the humanities, social, behavioral, and natural sciences?

Another issue that is rarely discussed is the question of whether the program is needed to meet local, state, or national needs. The initiation of any new program should take into account feasibility and need. I am skeptical about the need for so many baccalaureate programs in nursing. I suspect that many baccalaureate programs now in existence will close in the next ten years. Does the market exist for so many programs? Even more important, could not the profession achieve even greater momentum with a concentration of efforts and resources? We may face some intense criticism about the ineffective and inappropriate use of scarce resources.

My conclusion, then, after reviewing the nature of the models being developed and the many issues involved is that many of these programs do not possess the elements required for sound baccalaureate preparation in nursing. Full colleges and universities are essential to the achievement of professional baccalaureate nursing education.

NEED FOR LIBERAL EDUCATION

Nursing, like other professions, is an essential part of the society out of which it grew and with which it has been evolving. Nursing can be said to be owned by society, in the sense that nursing's professional interest must be perceived as serving the interest of the larger whole of which it is a part. In a recent article on the value of humanities in nursing, Donaldson nicely illustrates the blending of scientific knowledge and humanistic approach that ensures nursing's continued social relevance.[2] She points out that humanism is concerned with the growing realization of human potential. Humanists are all those who attempt to ameliorate the human condition. To seek knowledge for increasing human potential, nurses must know what human potential means. They must deal with such questions as who we are, what it means to be human, and what it means to live a human life. The answers to these questions vary considerably, just as the history of human culture varies in its style of expression, symbolism, and philosophy. Only through a broad liberal education do students of nursing learn to deal with some of these issues and gain a perspective and sensitivity so that they may assist individuals as various issues arise in response to common human predicaments.

---

[2] Sue Donaldson, "Let Us Not Abandon the Humanities," *Nursing Outlook* (January-February, 1983).

The profession of nursing must be committed to the continuance and enhancement of professional programs within the liberal education tradition. Liberal education is essential to the basics of nursing. Basic values gained through a sound preprofessional base in liberal education are highly valued in the profession. Individuals develop independent intelligence, leadership capacity, and adaptability, which provide benefits for the society as a whole. Individuals who have experienced liberal learning know how to deal with ambiguity and are capable of making responsible judgments about their own life and, in nursing, about the lives of others. Students of liberal education must acquire greater clarity of expression, read with greater understanding, and become literate, thinking, responsible citizens. They must understand the relationship among various branches of knowledge, which is essential to dealing with the scientific, applied, and humanistic components of nursing knowledge. They must possess the ability to transfer values in varied and complex situations.

The integrity of professional nursing education can only be assured if there is an appropriate relationship between liberal education and professional education. We must value association with liberal arts and work to have the appropriate balance between professional and liberal education to ensure appropriate quality in all program goals.

In a 1974 position paper for the American Association of Colleges of Nursing, Rogers stressed that knowledgeable practice in nursing is necessary, and full colleges and universities are essential to its achievement:

> The distinguishing characteristic of professional education in nursing is the transmission of nursing's body of abstract knowledge arrived at by scientific research and logical analysis—not a body of technical skills. This is not to deny the technical skills but rather to make clear that it is nursing's organized body of theoretical knowledge that identifies nursing as a profession. It is the utilization of this knowledge in service to people that determines the nature of nursing service. It is this body of knowledge which encompasses nursing's descriptive, explanatory, and predictive principles which guide its practitioners and make possible professional practice: A fulfillment of nursing's scientific humanitarianism.[3]

Professional education in nursing requires:

1. A full college or university.

2. An organizational structure for nursing that provides for full professional autonomy.

---

[3] Martha E. Rogers, "The Nature and Characteristics of Professional Education for Nursing" (Washington, D.C.: American Association of Colleges of Nursing, 1974).

3. A qualified nurse faculty.

4. Lower-division general education and appropriate upper-division cognate courses in the arts and sciences.

5. A substantive upper-division major in nursing characterized by the transmission of an organized body of scientific nursing knowledge.

6. Laboratory study whereby students have opportunity to translate theoretical knowledge in nursing into human service directed toward maintaining and promoting health and caring for and rehabilitating the sick and disabled.

7. Learning to exploit nursing knowledge for the improvement of the practice of nursing.

8. Acculturation of the student as a learned professional peer of other professional personnel.

9. Development of personal and professional accountability and responsible citizenship.

In March 1984, the membership of the American Association of Colleges of Nursing further articulated its beliefs in a position statement on single-purpose educational institutions:

> Professional education in nursing parallels that of the other professions and occurs in institutions of higher education. These institutions are characterized by instructional offerings in the arts, humanities, and sciences in a variety of disciplines, and by support systems for the socialization of the student into intellectual and investigative inquiry. They constitute a rich intellectual environment with multifaceted libraries, institutes, and centers and opportunities for integrative liberal learning with students from other disciplines and cultures, freedom of inquiry, and exploration into the wide realms of knowledge and values.
>
> The goals of institutions of higher learning have differed from those of single purpose institutions and have, by tradition and example, focused on bringing the fullest potential of mankind's cumulative intellect to the resolution of the dilemmas confronting the human condition. They provide for the development of the learner's ability to think for oneself, to master analytical problem solving, to apply scientific knowledge, and to make value judgements. The singular function of professional nursing is the improvement of the human condition. Education for the profession requires a broad academic orientation.[4]

Institutions assuming responsibility for professional baccalaureate nurs-

---

[4] "Single Purpose Institutions (Washington, D.C.: American Association of Colleges of Nursing, March 1984).

ing education are urged to carefully review the essential characteristics of higher education and baccalaureate education for nursing. In March 1985, the American Association of Colleges of Nursing will provide a list of qualified consultants to assist schools and colleges which are contemplating a transition to baccalaureate education in nursing.

Professional nursing organizations are not alone in their concern about what is occurring in baccalaureate education. The report of the Study Group on the Conditions of Excellence in American Higher Education was recently released.[5] A report on humanities in education, titled, "To Reclaim a Legacy," was also based on the study group's report.[6] The Association of American Colleges' book based on their project on redefining the meaning and purpose of baccalaureate degrees, *A Search for Quality and Coherence in Baccalaureate Education,* is highly recommended.[7]

In December 1983, the Association of American Colleges held a conference on the theme of "Integrating Liberal and Professional Education." In their attempt to develop a consensus about the topic, several principles of baccalaureate education were adopted, including the following:

1. Graduates of all baccalaureate programs should have certain characteristics in common that mark them as educated people, regardless of the type of undergraduate preparation.

2. Institutional and specialized accrediting agencies should promote discussions on the relationship between liberal and professional education in the baccalaureate degree program at their meetings.

3. Institutional and specialized accreditors need to emphasize the unity of all learning.

4. Institutional accrediting associations should take responsibility for helping colleges and universities to define the meaning of their baccalaureate degree.[8]

All these conferences and papers have dealt with the critical concern for quality in baccalaureate education. They identify essential and common characteristics of the baccalaureate degree program.

---

[5] Study Group on the Conditions of Excellence in American Higher Education, "Involvement in Learning: Realizing the Potential of American Higher Education," *Chronicle of Higher Education,* October 24, 1984, pp. 35–49.

[6] "To Reclaim a Legacy," *Chronicle of Higher Education,* November 28, 1984.

[7] *A Search for Quality and Coherence in Baccalaureate Education* (Washington, D.C.: Association of American Colleges, 1983).

[8] "Integrating Liberal and Professional Education" (Washington, D.C.: Association of American Colleges, 1983).

CONCLUSION

I urge that the nursing profession engage in careful analysis of the implications of actions planned today. We owe it to society to ensure the development of the best programs possible. Quality baccalaureate education in nursing requires a full college context, and we must make sure that whatever models we develop incorporate the essential components. The panel on excellence in education put it nicely, and although it is directed toward potential college students, there is a message for nursing in this statement as well:

> Over the next 15 years and into the next century, our nation will require citizens who have learned how to learn—who can identify, organize, and use all of the learning resources at their disposal. It will depend on creative people who can synthesize and reshape information and who can analyze problems from many different perspectives. And it will require people who will share their knowledge and intellectual abilities in family, community, and national life. Becoming one of those people will entail risks on your part. In all of our recommendations we have urged you to get as involved as you can in your own education—and getting involved is a risky business. Accept the challenge. The rewards are worth it.[9]

Nursing owes the society it serves quality baccalaureate programs that exist in full colleges and universities.

---

[9] Study Group on the Conditions of Excellence in American Higher Education, "Involvement in Learning."

A CASE FOR
THE SINGLE-PURPOSE
DEGREE-GRANTING COLLEGE
OF NURSING

SHARON E. BOLIN, MA, RN
Dean, West Suburban College of Nursing
Oak Park, Illinois

The issue of single-purpose degree-granting colleges of nursing has attracted much attention, if not notoriety, during the past few years. My purpose in this paper is to defend this concept as one which, if properly instituted, is educationally sound, comprising all the characteristics of baccalaureate nursing education that are embraced by mainstream thinking today.

In February 1981, the Board of Directors of the National League for Nursing adopted a "Position Statement on Preparation for Practice in Nursing." That statement reads, in part, "Educational programs in nursing must be adaptive and responsive to the nursing needs of the people, and must plan accordingly to prepare practitioners to meet these needs.... Experimentation and innovation in all programs will be necessary to attract sufficient numbers of practitioners at all levels and to prepare them to meet the nation's health care needs."

Some of us took the NLN Board of Directors seriously, and during the past few years experimentation has begun. The trend toward single-purpose degree-granting colleges of nursing has emerged. Although this phenomenon is new to nursing, it is well accepted in general education and other professional fields at both the undergraduate and graduate levels. According to Richard M. Millard, president of the Council on Postsecondary Accreditation:

There are currently at least ten fields in which there are free-standing professional institutions which are authorized legally to grant professional degrees and which are accredited. These are in the areas of art, chiropractic, law, medicine, music, osteopathy, pharmacy, podiatry, clinical psychology, and theology. They include some of the most prestigious institutions in the country in these fields.[1]

Millard further explains that "any institution that offers associate, baccalaureate, or advanced degrees is by definition a higher education institution." He disagrees with the position that "the only types of higher education institutions with the privilege of granting professional degrees are the complex higher education institutions," meaning the university.

There are at present several administrative models for single-purpose degree-granting colleges of nursing. One is the two-year, upper-division college of nursing, into which all students transfer when they have completed the equivalent of two years of prescribed liberal arts and sciences at the lower-division level. The degree is awarded by the college of nursing upon completion of two years of upper-division work in nursing. The second, and perhaps more prevalent model, is the freestanding college of nursing, which awards the degree jointly with a liberal arts college. There are also variations on these two themes. Since I am associated with a joint degree-granting program, this paper will focus on that model in particular.

A JOINT DEGREE PROGRAM

The administrative model for operation of the nursing program instituted by Concordia College in River Forest, Illinois, and the West Suburban College of Nursing in Oak Park, Illinois, is acknowleged by each institution to be a nontraditional, yet sound model. Each college is independent of the other organizationally and administratively, and each functions under its own board. However, the two schools are related contractually, and assume equal and joint responsibility for the baccalaureate nursing program.

The following underlying concerns were given serious attention in establishing the joint nursing program:

1. A strong liberal arts foundation should be the basis on which the nursing major is built.

2. Linkages between the two colleges should be planned and should occur at the organizational, administrative, faculty, and student levels.

3. Governance of the college of nursing should be by a college of nursing board, consisting of representation from the community at large.

---

[1] Quoted in "Excerpts from Responses to the AACN Position Paper on Single Purpose Institutions," *AACN Newsletter*, 10 (August 1984).

4. The financial future of the college of nursing should be secure, regardless of the fate of third-party reimbursement for nursing education.

5. The program must be established according to the accreditation criteria of both the regional accrediting body (the North Central Association in Illinois) and the National League for Nursing Council of Baccalaureate and Higher Degree Programs.

6. Students should be assured of entry into graduate programs in nursing upon graduation from this program.

Each of these points will be discussed in turn.

Liberal Arts Education

The faculties of both Concordia College and the West Suburban College of Nursing are committed to a liberal arts education for students. They believe that education from this perspective will produce a better prepared nurse and will improve the profession. The faculties believe that education in the liberal sense enables individuals to share knowledge and experience with others, particularly those whom they are serving, and that liberally educated professional nurses can do this. These nurses are able to articulate a broad view of social problems and can lead the client or clients to make their own health-related decisions in times of both wellness and illness. Significantly, they are better equipped to interpret the client to other health care professionals at a moment when clear communications are vital. Liberally educated nurses are further equipped with skills that enable them to think conceptually and to be effective learners, long after the formal education process has ended.

In the Concordia College–West Suburban College of Nursing program the general education requirements for nursing majors (humanities, fine arts, natural sciences, and social sciences) are determined by the faculty of Concordia College. These requirements are the same for other students seeking the baccalaureate degree at Concordia College, regardless of major. The general education courses that directly support the nursing major are jointly determined by the faculties of both colleges. The courses that make up the nursing major are determined by the faculty of the West Suburban College of Nursing. In this program, nursing courses begin during the sophomore year. Liberal arts courses continue throughout the program, with the equivalent of one upper-division liberal arts course taken during each quarter of the junior and senior years. This means that from the sophomore year on, students are taking courses on both campuses concurrently. This is in contrast to the model discarded by the profession many years ago, which sought to top off a diploma in nursing with two or three years of liberal arts courses at a college or university. The liberal arts courses were added on, not the foundation on which the nursing major was built, as they are in this program.

Linkages

Linkages between the two colleges have been built at the organizational, administrative, faculty, and student levels. The two colleges are united organizationally by a well-developed, highly detailed contract, which spells out individual and mutual obligations to students as well as other aspects of the program. The contract further requires that a coordinating committee, consisting of administrators of each of the institutions, meet at least quarterly to discuss and act on matters of concern to the joint nursing program. In addition, the dean of the West Suburban College of Nursing and the academic dean of Concordia College maintain a close working relationship. Arrangements have been and continue to be made for faculty members from each college to serve on faculty committees of the other college, and College of Nursing faculty participate fully in Concordia College's Fall Faculty Seminar. This ensures that the College of Nursing faculty have contact with faculty of other disciplines and that the faculty from Concordia College have interaction with the nursing faculty.

Linkages at the student level are considered to be of major importance. A liberal arts education takes place not only in the classroom, but in dormitory living and in cocurricular activities as well, and students should have natural opportunities for contacts at these levels. Nursing students are an integral part of almost every Concordia College cocurricular activity, including intra- and extramural sports and student government activities. Under the leadership of the first class of nursing students, a Nursing Student Organization was formed and has received formal recognition as a campus organization by the Student Council of Concordia College.

Students who are not commuters are required to live on Concordia's campus during the first two years of the program. Although the two schools are only a mile and a half apart, and a student-dispatched, student-driven van travels between the two campuses several times a day, both faculties believe that students should be in the mainstream of the liberal arts environment. When students become juniors, they have a choice of living on either campus. By that time they have had the opportunity to become well integrated into Concordia College campus life and have little difficulty finding their way back to that campus as they desire. To date, about one-third of the upper-class nursing students commute, one-third live at Concordia College, and one-third live at the College of Nursing. There is movement back and forth between residence halls on the two campuses during the year, depending on the preferences of the students.

Governance

Governance of the West Suburban College of Nursing is by the College of Nursing Board, whose primary concerns are the educational goals of the college and not those of the medical center of which it is a part. In its attempt to create such a structure, the college was directed by the North Central Association to the model used by an art museum containing an art institute. An art institute is an undergraduate, single-purpose, degree-granting institution of higher education, and it is also a legal entity of an art museum, a service organization. The chief executive officer of the art institute, the president, reports to the board of the art institute, which in turn is ultimately responsible to the board of the art museum. Likewise, the chief executive officer of the College of Nursing, the dean, reports to the College of Nursing Board, which in turn is responsible to the board of trustees of the medical center.

In keeping with this model, the corporate bylaws of the medical center were amended to create a College of Nursing Board, which comprises representation from the community at large. The seven-member board consists of the vice-chancellor of health affairs of a major university, the associate dean for graduate nursing education of a major Chicago university, the superintendent of a large public high school, the president of a steel merchandising business, the director of a dental health maintenance organization, a trustee of the medical center, and the chief executive officer of the medical center. The latter two board members may not be officers of the College of Nursing Board.

Third-Party Reimbursement

Prior to the establishment of the College of Nursing, the board of trustees of the medical center addressed the financial viability of the college, in the event that third-party reimbursement should become unavailable. They adopted the following resolution, dated June 22, 1981:

> Resolved, that the Board of Trustees continues to recognize the need for nurses prepared at the baccalaureate level and renews its commitment to the establishment and maintenance of a College of Nursing within the context of an academic climate consistent with traditional higher education, including allowances for academic freedom of both faculty and students with all the corresponding rights and responsibilities, and maintenance of an environment conducive to research, scholarship, and interdisciplinary exchange.
>
> Resolved, that the West Suburban Hospital Board of Trustees intends to maintain financial support for the College of Nursing should Medicare discontinue support of educational activities. Further resolved, that should this occur, alternate funding sources will be sought through the Development Department of the Medical Center and through community support.

It should be noted that a member of the College of Nursing Board has been appointed as a member of the board of the Development Foundation of the medical center in order to ensure attention to funding for the College of Nursing.

Accreditation

The program has been established according to accreditation criteria of both the North Central Association and the NLN Council of Baccalaureate and Higher Degree Programs. Concordia College is accredited by the North Central Association. The College of Nursing faculty wrote the self-study for candidacy with NCA during the 1983–84 academic year, had its site visit in April 1984, and was awarded candidacy status in August 1984. The first class of nursing students will graduate in May 1985, and the self-study for NCA accreditation of the College of Nursing will take place during the 1985–86 academic year. After that is accomplished, the program will be in a position to seek NLN accreditation.

Graduate Education

Concern for graduate education in nursing for graduates of this program was a consideration when the feasibility study was written for the Committee of Nursing Examiners of the Illinois Department of Registration and Education in 1981. The six colleges and universities in the greater Chicago area that have graduate programs in nursing were approached about whether students from this program would be accepted into their programs. All responded positively and indicated that their stipulations for graduates of programs not accredited by NLN would apply to graduates of this program until it achieved NLN accreditation.

TAKING THE STEP

The faculties of both Concordia College and the West Suburban College of Nursing recognize that we have taken a professional step that ultimately will be validated only by our product. We have attempted to demonstrate the spirit of creativity and innovation in the development of this baccalaureate nursing program, with an underlying commitment to educational integrity and academic freedom. I have been inspired by the words of Daniel Burnham, that great Chicago architect of the nineteenth century, who said:

> Make no Little Plans; they have no magic to stir men's blood and probably themselves will not be realized. Make Big Plans; aim high in hope and work, remembering that a noble, logical diagram once recorded will never die, but long after we are gone will be a living thing, asserting itself with evergrowing insistency. Remember that

our sons and grandsons are going to do things that would stagger us. Let your watchword be order and your beacon beauty.[2]

We have made big plans and are now implementing them. We are confident that the step that we took *will* be validated as a viable paradigm to be emulated in the future.

---

[2] Daniel H. Burnham, "Introduction," in Burnham and Edward H. Bennet, *Plan of Chicago* (New York: Da Capo Press, 1970), p. v.

A DISEASE CALLED 'EGALITARIANISM': SINGLE-PURPOSE INSTITUTIONS FOR NURSING

JULIA A. LANE, PhD, RN,
Dean, Marcella Niehoff School of Nursing
Loyola University of Chicago
Chicago, Illinois

For the last five years I have been increasingly discouraged over the inability of the nursing profession to speak with one voice about educational preparation and practice issues. My concern is epitomized in the phrase, "Egalitarianism, a disease from which professional nursing will die." Egalitarianism is the notion that everyone and every idea is equal, and the good of the profession is made subservient to this belief.

My concern is also embodied in the question: Can baccalaureate education for nursing be achieved in a single-purpose institution? "Single-purpose institution," in this instance, is a euphemism for a hospital school of nursing. It is my belief that it cannot be done, and to propose that it can be done is to confuse essence with function. The confusing of essence with function has been a problem perpetuated within the profession of nursing for the past two decades. Arendt described it when she wrote: "I am confused when I call the heel of my shoe a hammer because I, like most women, use it to drive a nail into a wall."[1] We are confused when we believe an institution whose essence is a hospital school can call itself a college and thus become one.

My thesis is that a single-purpose institution cannot (1) offer the essence

---

[1] Hannah Arendt, *Between Past and Future* (New York: Viking Press, 1966), p. 102.

of a college education, (2) advance the goals of the nursing profession, (3) meet the criteria set forth by the profession for baccalaureate education, or (4) promote the image of nursing as a professional discipline. Obtaining a state charter and candidacy from a regional accrediting body does not guarantee that an institution will achieve the hallmarks of a college. A college, as an institution of higher learning, is more than the sum of its parts.

THE NATURE OF A COLLEGE

What is a college? Traditionally, it is defined as a self-governing society of scholars who come together for the purpose of study and instruction—a community of scholars engaged in teaching and research. The chief goal of the college and university is to train and develop the human intellect, extending the power of independent and balanced thought and deepening the power of discrimination and critical expression.[2]

What should a student expect of a college? Educators agree on four main points:[3]

1. Students should acquire a positive and realistic conception of their abilities in the world of higher learning and in the world at large. Therefore, they need a diversity of experience and associates to achieve this self-awareness.

2. Students should reach the point of being able to see the structure and interrelations of knowledge in order to begin the process of forming judgments on their own. Therefore, they need faculty and a milieu that demonstrates the interrelationships in their daily life and their professional discipline.

3. Students should see the relevance of higher education to the quality of their own life. Therefore, they need models who demonstrate the relevance of a broad range of knowledge to enrich human development and enhance life's satisfaction.

4. Students should expect to prepare for work.

A recent report of the Study Group on the Conditions of Excellence in American Higher Education states: ''The student outcomes should not only include knowledge, intellectual capacity and skills but dimensions of student growth such as self confidence, persistence, leadership, empathy, social responsibility and understanding of cultural and intellec-

[2] *The Student in Higher Education,* report of the Committee in Higher Education (Connecticut: The Hogan Foundation, 1968), p. 8.

[3] *Ibid.,* p. 10.

tual differences.[4] To achieve these outcomes requires an appropriate milieu, faculty, and resources. The report goes on to say that higher education will mean little if the degrees the students seek are weakened as a credential by reduced standards, if academic institutions offer vocational curricula, or it they allow academic credentials to supersede the pursuit of learning or accepted definitions of quality. This is the issue we face today.

THE ESSENCE OF COLLEGE EDUCATION

My thesis is that a single-purpose institution cannot offer the essence of college education. I have reviewed the descriptive materials of five nursing programs based in single-purpose institutions. The five schools reviewed use different models. Four of them are affiliated with private, liberal arts colleges whose student enrollment is generally less than 1,500. One program is in a denominational teachers' college where the only bachelor of science degree offered is in nursing. The president of one program told me that she used the Rush model as the educational paradigm, although I saw no evidence that the school offered any other discipline. To a greater or lesser extent, the curriculum structures of these five institutions use the models that were in vogue between colleges and hospital schools in an earlier generation. These models were discontinued because it was felt that administration, environmental milieu, curriculum quality, and resource utilization were not centered in a single agent and hence were operationally ineffective in obtaining the objectives of a college education.

One hundred years ago, Newman recognized the value of the educational milieu:

> When a multitude of young men, keen and open-minded, sympathetic and observant, . . . come together and freely mix with each other, they are sure to learn from one another. . . . The conversation of all is a series of lectures to each and they gain for themselves new ideas and views, fresh matters of thought and distinct principles for judging and acting.[5]

Research also demonstrates that students' interactions with their teachers, their encounters with the social structure of college administration, the friendship groups in which they become integrated, the values they acquire from the student culture all have an immense if not precisely measured impact on the evolution of young people's view of self and

---

[4] Study Group on the Conditions of Excellence in American Higher Education, "Involvement in Learning: Realizing the Potential of American Higher Education," *Chronicle of Higher Education*, October 24, 1984, p. 37.

[5] John Henry Newman, *The Idea of University*, ed. Martin J. Svaglic, S.J. (New York: Rinehart & Co., 1960), p. 110.

world, on their confidence and altruism, and on their mastery of the need for identity.[6]

It is based on such an understanding of the nature and objectives of higher education that I state that the single-purpose institution is unable to offer the essence of a college education because it is unable to provide the milieu, the faculty, and resources demanded. I will address each of these factors individually.

Environmental Milieu

What milieu do we have in a single-purpose institution? The student's teachers are nurses, the social structure of administration is nursing, the friendship groups are nurses, the values are from nursing, the student culture is nursing, the environment itself is nursing. Will not the student's view of the world, the student's confidence, the student's identity be molded and controlled by nursing? Nursing education entered the academy to produce an educated person who has a sense of his or her own capacity with and against peers in a variety of disciplines. Can students from a single-purpose institution achieve this? How will these students perceive themselves—as educated individuals or as nurses? My hunch is that students will perceive themselves first as nurses, not as college graduates, because the environment essential to acquiring the self-concept of an educated person is not provided within a single-purpose institution.

Faculty

What of the faculty in a single-purpose institution? Do they see themselves as academic faculty? Do they have the qualifications of other academic faculty? Are they engaged in scholarly activities? Do faculty share in the governance of the affiliated institutions? Even though several of the schools I reviewed offered a joint degree, faculty of the nursing college were listed in an appendix in the catalogs and not integrated into the affiliated college faculty roster.

Can faculty who are not themselves part of the academic environment impart an academic environment? I believe that they cannot, yet faculty and students are the essence of college life. Unless faculty develop the milieu appropriate to higher education, the essence of a college cannot exist no matter how it functions.

Resources

As a result of limited student enrollment, a single-purpose institution will not be able to provide the resources needed to maintain a quality

[6] Study Group on the Conditions of Excellence in American Higher Education, "Involvement in Learning," p. 6.

program. It is fairly certain that the current subsidization of hospital-linked nursing education by Medicare, Medicaid, and third-party payers will be eliminated. Furthermore, it is predicted that many more small colleges in the United States will close due to a shrinking pool of students and shrinking financial resources. It is these portents of the future, I believe, that prompted Rodgers to say: "We do not know...whether or not the marriages that force and circumstances are currently fastening between hospital schools and other post-secondary educational institutions, will prove to be compatible and long lived or end in messy divorces."[7]

GOALS OF NURSING

A single-purpose institution does not advance the goal of professional nursing, which has been and is to place nursing within institutions of higher education. In 1876, Abby Woolsey stressed the desirability of elevating nursing to an educated profession.[8] She believed that nursing schools should be within the mainstream of higher education. This belief was reiterated by Goldmark in 1923, Goodrich in 1932, Brown in 1948, and by the American Nurses' Association's position paper on education in 1965 and resolution on baccalaureate education in 1978.[9] Nowhere have nursing leaders or the profession suggested that we begin our own institutions! Furthermore, the intent of the shift to higher education was not to produce better nurses, but to develop people who possesed a broad educational foundation received from the humanities and biophysical and behavioral sciences, people whose education would enhance them as individuals first and secondarily as nurses.

The advent of single-purpose institutions as the academy for nursing denigrates the hundred-year effort of the profession to place nursing education squarely within the realm of higher education.

Hospital schools have long fought the ANA's 1965 position paper and 1978 resolution reaffirming baccalaureate entry into the profession. Is not the miraculous conversion of hospital schools toward higher education in 1984 rooted in the economics of declining student enrollments, not ideology? Although all schools of nursing are affected by drops in

[7] Bernard F. Rodgers, Jr., "Educational Mobility for Hospital Schools of Nursing," paper presented at the American Hospital Association Conference, Chicago, March 17–18, 1983.

[8] Abby Woolsey, *A Century of Nursing,* cited in *A Case for Baccalaureate Preparation in Nursing* (Kansas City, Mo: American Nurses Association, 1979).

[9] Josephine Goldmark, *A Study of Nursing and Nursing Education in the United States,* report of the Committee for the Study of Nursing Education (New York: Macmillan Co. 1932); Annie W. Goodrich, "The School of Nursing and the Future," in *Proceedings of the Thirty-Eighth Annual Convention of the National League of Nursing Education* (New York: National League of Nursing Education, 1932), p. 173; and Esther Lucille Brown, *Nursing for the Future,* report prepared for the National Nursing Council (New York: Russell Sage Foundation, 1948), p. 77.

enrollment, diploma schools are affected to a greater extent because of society's emphasis on a college education. Moreover, I suspect that a key variable in the support for single-purpose institutions by some nurse faculty is job security.

Therefore, I maintain that the creation of single-purpose schools of nursing was not the intent of the profession, nor will it forward the goals of the profession. Instead, it will weaken the very concept of baccalaureate education for nursing and act as an impediment to future professional development.

STANDARDS FOR EDUCATION

Single-purpose institutions do not meet the ANA standards for nursing education or the criteria of the National League for Nursing Council of Baccalaureate and Higher Degree Programs for accreditation. ANA's *Standards for Nursing Education* specify that the sponsoring institution must offer degrees in several disciplines.[10] The professional society also has specific standards for faculty and administration. I acknowledge my limited knowledge of the curriculum of the programs under discussion, but I have serious reservation about the curriculum of one multiple-exit program in which the diploma graduate and baccalaureate graduate have the same educational courses.

In relation to NLN criteria, my concern is how the single-purpose institution defines the "parent" institution and how the affiliated college institution relates to the single-purpose institutions in regard to structure, governance, faculty, resources, and policies.[11] I suspect an interlocking directorship through the hospital as the "parent institution." In one single-purpose institution, the structure is fairly obvious because the chief executive officer of the hospital corporation writes the introduction to the catalog.

The course titles and course offerings in some single-purpose programs appear appropriate, although numerous, suggesting an imbalance between nursing and general studies. For example, in one program there are only 21 total credit hours of general education and 18 credit hours of science education in 150 credit hours needed for the degree. Yet, the report on the Conditions of Excellence in American Higher Education cited earlier stressed the need of professional students, including those in nursing, for a grounding in a liberal and general education if they are to provide truly professional service to their clients.[12]

From my assessment, therefore, I believe that a single-purpose institution does not meet the criteria for academic and professional ac-

---

[10] *Standards for Nursing Education* (Kansas City, Mo.: American Nurses' Association, 1975).

[11] Council of Baccalaureate and Higher Degree Programs, *Self-Study Manual: Guidelines for Preparation of the Self-Study Report* (New York: National League for Nursing, 1984).

[12] Study Group on the Conditions of Excellence in Higher Education, "Involvement in Learning."

creditation. However, I leave this decision to a jury of my peers on the board of review.

THE IMAGE OF NURSING

My final point is that a single-purpose institution cannot promote the image of nursing as a professional discipline. A professional discipline by its nature, must be located squarely within the university. For a century, nursing has struggled to move its image toward professional status. Professional status is obtained initially through education.

What message are we giving to the consumer about the professional status of nursing education when a hospital school can call itself a college without meeting the usual attributes implied by the word? What message is given to physicians, to legislature, to patients, to other disciplines? Can they really believe that we are professionals?

Styles has said that "a profession that does not believe in anything cannot achieve excellence."[13] What does nursing believe in? Will not single-purpose institutions in nursing education devalue the whole process of education for nursing for their own self-preservation?

CONCLUSION

A nursing educator with a sense of history, an open mind, and a knowledge of the trends affecting our programs can see the problems we face. We have permitted colleges with no interest in nursing education to use nurses to increase their enrollments by offering them professional degrees without upper-division nursing majors. The sad part of this state of affairs is seen in the nurses who naively enroll in these programs.

We have seen people enter professional nursing through competency examinations from programs without supervised clinical practice. Now we see the newest aberration—hospital schools calling themselves colleges. At some point we must stand collectively, state what we believe in, and act on it. If we refuse to act as gatekeepers for our professional standards, as medicine and law have traditionally done, then we shall die of the disease called "egalitarianism." If that happens...may we rest in peace. Nobody killed us. We did it to ourselves.

---

[13] M. Styles, "Fiftieth Anniversary Address," Loyola University of Chicago, Chicago, Illinois, October 1984 (mimeographed).

ASSESSING SINGLE-PURPOSE INSTITUTIONS THROUGH THE ACCREDITATION PROCESS

SHARON L. DIAZ, RN, MS
President, Samuel Merritt College of Nursing
Oakland, California

The aim of this paper is not to advocate or defend single-purpose degree-granting institutions of higher education. Such institutions have been an integral part of higher education throughout its history and evolution. Law, theology, engineering, music, and medicine are among the professions thus educated. Therefore, the question, it would seem, is not the role of the single-purpose institution in higher education, or even, I suspect, in baccalaureate degree nursing education. The real issues lie with the essence of baccalaureate degree nursing education and the fear that the current development of single-purpose, degree-granting institutions in nursing will, at a minimum, diminish the hard-won progress of the last 20 years and, at worst, relegate nursing education to the bleakness of the years preceding 1950.

To address this fear, I am compelled to address what I think people believe but aren't saying: that a medical center or conceivably a single hospital is an inappropriate sponsor to a baccalaureate degree nursing program. Once again, I must urge closer scrutiny of institutional models of higher education. Not every college and university is the "natural child" of its parent. Vintners, automakers, institutes for policy studies, and, some might argue, church and state make unlikely sponsors of colleges and universities, but they are. Therefore, I am inclined to conclude that the issue is really not who the parent is, but rather how she parents.

66 □ SHARON L. DIAZ

How then might one qualitatively assess the single-purpose degree-granting institution in nursing? My simplistic answer is: Use the existing system. By that I mean the accrediting processes that have withstood and evolved through many trials.

REGIONAL ACCREDITATION

Generally, state regulations set minimum standards for degree-granting institutions. The regional accreditation process, however, is specifically designed to determine if an institution, whether single-purpose or general, meets the qualitative standards expected of institutions of higher education—standards and criteria developed by peer institutions that reflect the values and expertise of their representatives. This qualitative self-study and review process is comprehensive in depth and breadth from an institutional rather than a program perspective.

During 1983 and 1984, the Samuel Merritt College of Nursing underwent this process, devoting 18 months to intensive and extensive self-study by representatives of all members of the college community. The entire process—the self-study, the four-day site visit by a six-member team (including two nurse educators), and the commission review—was developmental and facilitative, promoting awareness of institutional strengths and weaknesses and providing direction for planned institutional change and improvement. As the self-study evolved, and in consultation with staff of the Western Association of Schools and Colleges, it became apparent that the college was prepared to seek full accreditation rather than candidacy status. Indeed, the Senior Commission of the Western Association of Schools and Colleges acted in June to confer the maximum five-year, full initial accreditation to the College of Nursing.

Once regionally accredited, a single-purpose degree-granting institution is eligible to seek voluntary specialized accreditation of its educational program. Such programs in nursing should be assessed against existing criteria that reflect key elements and characteristics of baccalaureate degree nursing education. Special criteria and policies need not be developed to assess this nontraditional approach to baccalaureate degree nursing education any more than they were needed during the evolution of the "second-step," RN-baccalaureate degree programs and external degree programs.

Within the context of the existing criteria, however, are critical issues for single-purpose institutions that need particular scrutiny. These are (1) Can such institutions provide a curriculum that embodies the essence—the philosophy, goals, and resources—of baccalaureate nursing education? and (2) Can they demonstrate a financial and philosophical commitment to education as a primary mission? It is appropriate that these issues be addressed within the established professional accreditation process.

As is apparent, some schools have successfully followed the recommendation of the 1970 Lysaught report of the National Commission for the Study of Nursing and Nursing Education that "those hospital schools that are strong and vital, endowed with a qualified faculty, suitable educational facilities and motivated for excellence be encouraged to seek and obtain regional accreditation and degree-granting power."[1] How many more will be successful in doing so, and how they will change the face of nursing education, I cannot predict. As Clark Kerr has stated in *More Than Survival,* "It takes a dash of bravado to make a projection; but a touch of madness to believe too much in its invincibility."[2]

I believe, however, that the development of various institutional models will have little ultimate impact and that this "movement" will not take the country by storm. Supporting this view are existing quality controls and current realities regarding costs and sources of financial support for higher education, including nursing education.

As noted, the regional accreditation process serves as a mechanism for institutional quality control—assessing such characteristics as institutional purposes; integrity; governance and administration; educational programs; faculty and staff; student services; and learning, physical, and financial resources. The professional accreditation process, then, provides for the evaluation of the program against criteria that are believed to define quality baccalaureate nursing education.

The resources required for a diploma school to successfully complete a rebirth into a degree-granting institution are phenomenal. Sound, careful, and extensive planning, coupled with an organizational milieu too complex to describe here, require far more than mere financial support. However, the implementation of diagnosis-related groups (DRGs) and the elimination of reimbursement mechanisms for medical and nursing education sponsored by hospitals will cause further diminution in the number and, in some cases, quality of diploma programs. These changes in financing will also act to inhibit their evolution to degree-granting institutions.

DIVERSITY AND INNOVATION

In conclusion, I would raise two points. First, one does not draw a scientifically valid conclusion based upon an assessment of one

[1] National Commission for the Study of Nursing and Nursing Education, J. P. Lysaught, director, *An Abstract for Action* (New York: McGraw-Hill Book Co., 1970), p. 109.

[2] Carnegie Foundation for the Advancement of Teaching, *More Than Survival: Prospects for Higher Education in a Period of Uncertainty* (San Francisco: Jossey-Bass, 1975).

characteristic of the phenomenon under study. The institutional setting of a baccalaureate degree nursing program is but one of many important characteristics. Second, higher education and higher education in nursing have not reached their current levels of excellence through homogeneity, but rather through a philosophy that values diversity and innovation.

Building a
Knowledge Base

DIALECTICS OF
THEORY DEVELOPMENT

PATRICIA MOCCIA, PhD, RN
Associate Professor, School of Nursing
College of New Rochelle
New Rochelle, New York

Dialectics as a philosophy is concerned with a reality that is characterized by an incessant process of change and transformation. Dialectics
as a method of inquiry searches to uncover, identify, and assign
significance to the *relationships* between the parts of any system and the
relationships between parts and the totality. Dialectics as a method of
exposition is especially concerned with design and data display, emphasiz-
ing the changes that have occurred in the process of investigation from
the original conceptualizations of the problem, through the data collection and tentative findings, to the analytical phases. Dialectics as a process of intellectual reconstruction pays special attention to integrating
newly discovered understandings into the original thoughts on the problem, acknowledging the whys and wherefores of what has *changed* since
the question under consideration was first posed. Finally, dialectics as
a dialectical process necessarily includes the transforming relationships
between these four definitions as a world view, as a method of inquiry,
as a method of exposition and as a process of intellectual reconstruction.[1]

Given the richness of such a definition, dialectics has a full and comprehensive potential for theory development in nursing. First, there are
the possibilities that dialectics might serve to unite several conceptual
models without compromising their uniqueness (perhaps in the way a

---

[1] Bertell Ollman, *Alienation: Marx's Conception of Man in Capitalist Society* (2nd ed; Cambridge, England:
Cambridge University Press, 1976), p. 52.

"disciplinary matrix" would, as Fawcett has described).[2] In addition, the dialectic holds special promise for two specific questions that are currently debated in the literature. The first we share with other disciplines—that is, how to accommodate and reconcile the differences between qualitative and quantitative approaches to research. The second is unique to our discipline—how, if at all, to study holistic processes, such as human phenomena, or contingent ones such as relational interactions, with particulate methods.

DIALECTICS

Dialectics, as defined in this discussion, is consistent with the general understanding of the dialectic. It is a world view that assumes that the basic unit of life is a totality; that this totality or system is characterized by a constant process of self-transformation; that this incessant change is generated by and developed through the interrelationships among the totality's parts; and that these interrelationships are themselves dynamic.[3]

Obviously, dialectics has other potentials than the three already identified, including a potential to confuse. Dialectics can be confusing, first because of its multidimensional, multifaceted nature. Second, there are predictable misunderstandings that result when different authors or, in some cases, the same author in different places, uses the term without clarifying which of its particular aspects they are addressing.

In addition, an equally predictable confusion has developed because of the dialectic's remarkable long and varied philosophical history. As a metaphysics concerned with being as process and movement it can be traced to Anaximander (c. 611–547 BC) and Aristotle (384–322 BC); as a method of investigation it dates back to Socrates and Plato (c. 428–348 BC). More recently, the dialectic has been enjoying a popular revival in both the natural and social sciences, being used in disciplines as seemingly different as astronomy, physics, chemistry, biology, psychology, and sociology.[4]

There is yet another factor, neither as predictable nor as understandable, contributing to the confusion surrounding the dialectic. There seems to be an almost phobic aversion to the considerable amount of work in this area by German philosophers Georg Wilhelm Hegel and Karl Marx and an apparently facile dismissal of either their relevance or significance. There is no argument with the fact that these philosophers have some very strong critics. (Popper, for example, has called Hegel's

---

[2] J. Fawcett, "The Metaparadigm of Nursing: Present Status and Future Refinements," *Image*, 16, No. 3 (Summer 1984), p. 85.

[3] D. D. Runes, ed., *Dictionary of Philosophy* (Totowa, N.J.: Littlefield, Adams & Co., 1975).

[4] K. F. Riegel, "The Dialectics of Human Development," *American Psychologist* (1976), pp. 689–700.

dialectic "bombastic and mystifying cant."[5]) Nevertheless, Hegel and Marx are considered by many as two of the three great philosophers of modern thought (Kierkegaard being the third).[6] And yet, the Hegelian-Marxist dialectic has been either ignored without any obvious reason or, in some cases, discounted on the basis of the subsequent political ideologies developed by these philosophers.[7] This is comparable to Democrats in this country refusing forevermore to watch any television because Ronald Reagan has perfected the use of the medium for political propaganda.

Dialectics, as developed by Hegel, Marx, or others working in the tradition of either or both, deserves the attention of nursing scholars for several reasons—*most importantly because the world views of both Hegel and Marx are consistent with nursing's concerns,* at a time when finding compatible world views has become a frustrating, if not exasperating, endeavor. Hegel developed his system from the understanding that being is a universal process of constant movement. He goes on to postulate that "The truth is the whole. The whole, however, is merely the essential nature reaching its completeness through the process of its own becoming."[8] Nature is defined as a process of negation, whereby a creative dynamic force unites with what seems to be its own contradiction and so forms a unity or what is recognized as the whole.

Marx differs from Hegel on several significant points, which are beyond this discussion. He held fast, however, to Hegel's theoretical foundations of (1) being as a constant process of transformation, and (2) the dialectical nature of this ongoing change.[9] And while the historical lineage of dialectics becomes increasingly circuitous, Hegelian and Marxist dialecticians identify themselves by a necessary adherence to these two principles. The dialectic of this paper, as defined by Ollman, continues in this tradition of Hegel and Marx.[10]

---

[5] Karl R. Popper, *The Open Society and Its Enemies,* Vol. 2: *The High Tide of Prophecy: Hegel, Marx and the Aftermath* (5th ed; Princeton, N.J.: Princeton University Press, 1971.), p. 28.

[6] R. Heiss, *Hegel, Kierkegaard, Marx: Three Great Philosophers Whose Ideas Changed the Course of Civilization,* trans. E. B. Garside (New York: Dell Publishing Co., 1975), p. x.

[7] L. M. Wilson and J. J. Fitzpatrick, "Dialectical Thinking as a Means of Understanding Systems-in-Development: Relevance to Rogers's Principles," *Advances in Nursing Science,* 6, No. 2 (1984), p. 31.

[8] Georg W. Hegel, *The Phenomenology of Mind,* trans. J. B. Baillie (London: Allen & Unwin, 1964), p. 55.

[9] Karl Marx, *Grundrisse: Foundations of the Critique of Political Economy,* trans. M. Nicolaus (New York: Vintage Books, 1973), p. 90.

[10] Ollman, *Alienation.*

VALUE OF DIALECTICS AS METHOD

Quantitative or Qualitative?

A second reason Hegelian-Marxist dialectics deserves our attention is because of the consistency between its world view and its method of inquiry, and the value of such consistency to nurse researchers. With increasing frequency, scholars are questioning the adequacy and appropriateness of researching nursing's concerns with quantitative methodologies.[11] Whether nursing's concerns are defined as a human life process characterized as holistic, dynamic, and/or developmental (which is occurring in a growing number of conceptual frameworks) or as people relating to each other and their environments (which has historically been the case), the debate focuses on whether or not the constraints imposed by the principles of scientific experimentation generate information of such specificity and discreteness as to have little, if any, usefulness to theorizing about nursing's holistic or relational concerns.

In addition to such practical concerns, another aspect of the questioning focuses on whether greater attention should be paid to assuring that there is an internal coherence to nursing's metaparadigm. These arguments are developed from the assumptions that nursing's world view, its values, and its analytical tools should show a degree of congruence not found when nursing concerns are approached from within the prevailing scientific paradigm. And so, scholars turn to qualitative methods such as phenomenology, grounded theories, feminist paradigms, or dialectics as more appropriate, given parallels between their foci, values, and interests and those of nursing.

There is, however, a difficulty with using qualitative methods, as currently developed, to study nursing's concerns, which is recognized by even their most ardent supporters. The problem that develops when using such methods is their inadequacy in providing information necessary for nursing to predict and control the phenomena under study. Attempts to resolve such inadequacies usually try to synthesize quantitative and qualitative approaches at either the theoretical or practical levels. So, for example, phenomenologists argue (and rightly so, given the limits

---

[11] K. I. MacPherson, "Feminist Methods: A New Paradigm for Nursing Research," *Advances in Nursing Science*, 5 (1983), pp. 17–25; P. L. Munhall, "Nursing Philosophy and Nursing Research: In Apposition or Opposition? *Nursing Research*, 31, No. 1 (1982), pp. 176–177ff; C. Oiler, "The Phenomenological Approach in Nursing Research," *Nursing Research*, 31, No. 3 (1982), pp. 178–181; A. Omery, "Phenomenology: A Method for Nursing Research," *Advances in Nursing Science*, 5 (1983), pp. 49–63; M. C. Silva and D. Rothbart, "An Analysis of Changing Trends in Philosophies of Science on Nursing Theory Development and Testing," *Advances in Nursing Science*, 6, No. 2 (1984), pp. 1–13; J. M. Swanson and W. C. Chenitz, "Why Qualitative Research in Nursing?" *Nursing Outlook*, 30, No. 4(1982), pp. 241–245; and M. B. Tinkle and J. L. Beaton, "Toward a New View of Science: Implications for Nursing Research," *Advances in Nursing Science*, 5 (1983), pp. 27–36.

of the approach) for their descriptive method as a complement to rather than an alternative to quantitative research.[12] Others argue for a synthesis or convergence approach that is both flexible and creative in its attempts to preserve the best of both worlds by placing a "new emphasis on contextual variables."[13]

As mentioned before, nursing is not alone in its struggles with this dilemma. Educational researchers, as one other example, are seeking to resolve what seems to be irreconcilable differences as they refine their study of the context and contingencies of social relationships with methods that produce both valid and verifiable information. A recent analysis suggests that researchers, in fact, are blending the two approaches in practice by increasing the uniformity and specificity of the ways they verify qualitative data.[14] While such a pragmatic solution has the potential to dissolve some of the differences between the two approaches by making qualitative data more like quantitative, it leads to the equivocal conclusions one can expect when the differences between world views are not addressed directly.

Such accommodations counter the original argument based on the inconsistencies between nursing's concerns and microscopic examination and pose their own internal contradictions that must be addressed. Either nursing's foci are holistic phenomena and relational processes or they are not. If not, then nursing research can continue to particularize, to measure and predict, contriving to fit people into models. However, if nursing insists on dynamic, developmental, and synergistic foci, it will have to find a way to deal with a "macroscopic imperative" that is a function of the irreducibility of such phenomena. Nursing's choice then becomes either (1) to study with internally inconsistent tools, which will lead to the original discrepancies; (2) to give up study altogether, which will call its social contract into question; or (3) to somehow accommodate to the "macroscopic imperative" by proceeding with a recognition of the inherent limits of any understanding and by exploiting such limits for the information they can provide about the larger system.

Dialectics—with its philosophy of incessant transformation—allows nursing to remain concerned with either holistic phenomena, contingent relationships, or both. With the congruence between its world view and its methods of study and exposition, dialectics provides nursing with ways to fulfill its social contract of expanding and refining its unique body of knowledge. And with its provisions for developmental relationships between its phases, the dialectic allows nursing a measure of internal

[12] Oiler, "The Phenomenological Approach in Nursing Research."

[13] L. D. Goodwin and W. L. Goodwin, "Qualitative vs. Quantitative Research or Qualitative *and* Quantitative Research? *Nursing Research,* 33 (November–December 1984), pp. 378–380.

[14] M. B. Miles and A. M. Huberman, "Drawing Valid Meaning from Qualitative Data: Toward a Shared Craft," *Educational Researcher* (May 1984), pp. 20–30.

coherence not found in past attempts to match methods to phenomena or, as more usually happens, to mold the phenomena to available methods. How it does so is discussed in the next section.

Individuation and Abstraction

Although a growing number of nursing scholars are concerned with a holistic life process, none is more insistent on its synergistic character than Rogers. Repeatedly and consistently, Rogers reminds us that "the whole is more than and different from the sum of its parts"; that "a field has meaning *only* in its entirety"; and that "the whole cannot be understood when it is reduced to its particulars."[15]

But even Rogers has to allow for divisions within the whole, as when she discusses boundaries between human and environmental fields. Defined by Rogers as energy fields that are coextensive with each other and the universe and, therefore, extend to infinity, the human and environmental fields are, nonetheless, divided by boundaries. These boundaries are arbitrary constructs and, most important in relation to the internal consistency of Rogers's discussion, are themselves constantly changing. While such an understanding gives Rogers and others concerned with holistic phenomena a theoretical window on how to approach study, it falls short of providing the boost through.

Dialectics also faces the seemingly impossible situation of studying a totality by necessarily reducing it to its parts (even if the parts are as broadly designed and as comprehensive as are the divisions of human and environmental fields) which, in the process, changes the original phenomena. The conceptual solution embraced by dialectics—which holds similar promise for nursing scholarship—is to (1) acknowledge the necessity of such divisions and its unavoidable distortion, and (2) study the distortion for what it can reveal about the underlying processes.

The activity of dividing the whole of the ongoing process of change and becoming into subunits or parts of the whole is defined within dialectics as the process of individuation. As Ollman discusses it, individuation is "simply a matter of mentally carving up the whole in a different manner for a particular purpose."[16] (How simple a matter it is would undoubtedly be debated by both beginning and more experienced researchers who are struggling to determine just what their variables really are.) These "particular purposes" are the "arbitrary boundaries" of Rogers's system and can include an individual's own needs or experiences, apparent similarities or contradictions within the phenomena,

[15] Martha E. Rogers, *An Introduction to the Theoretical Basis of Nursing* (Philadelphia: F. A. Davis Co., 1970), pp. 43–48, 89–94.

[16] Ollman, *Alienation*, p. 19.

seemingly similar or contrasting problems, or an inherent characteristic of the "human condition."[17] In any event, the significant points are that (1), despite the division, there continues to be contingent, transforming relationships between the parts and the whole; and (2) a dialectical study shifts the interest from the particular individuations or categories to the ongoing relational process between the units and the totality.

While obviously most helpful as a way out of a theoretical paradox, the process of individuation is not without conceptual and practical dangers. The most critical problem is attributed to the "forces of abstraction" whereby parts are perceived as the whole rather than as particular forms or manifestations of the whole.[18] When abstractions develop unacknowledged, individuations become increasingly distorted until there are layers and layers of parts masquerading as the whole, perceptions of reality becomes foggier and foggier, and the chances for accurate understanding are lost.

In general, then, individuations are most helpful when they are studied in relation to the whole and not as isolated phenomena. The abuse of the work of Freud is an example of the exponential distortions that emerge when a part is treated as a whole. The brilliant conceptualization of the unconscious promises people the opportunity to know their reality more fully. Its potential power is corrupted, however, when the unconscious is treated, not as a part of a process or as one aspect of reality, but instead as the sole reality that shapes and predetermines people's behavior. Such a misunderstanding of the unconscious robs people of the dynamic, creative interactions that distinguish their human nature. How markedly and productively different is an unconscious that is seen as one phase in the process of becoming.

Dialectics, through its subconcepts of individuation and abstraction, provides nurse scholars with constructs appropriate for the study of holistic phenomena, which do not ignore any "macroscopic imperative." Investigations that attempt to emphasize the relationships among the parts and between the parts and the whole are, in fact, more consistent with a holistic approach than are those that totally devalue particulate knowledge. By taking into account the processes of change and internal relations as two of the identifying characteristics of holistic phenomena, the dialectic validates a certain significance for both particulate knowledge and discrete measurements. For, within a system such as holism that recognizes an inherent developmental process of internal relations, knowledge—however limited or individuated—is itself always changing. And when a part's relationship to the whole is correctly identified as a developmental stage in a process of knowing the whole, then that

---

[17] *Ibid.*
[18] *Ibid.*

knowledge in some way illuminates the totality. So, rather than distracting from an understanding of the totality, individuated knowledge can uncover more of the underlying developmental process.

SUMMARY AND CONCLUSIONS

Thanks to the tremendous amount of work accomplished by nursing scholars over the last 10 to 20 years, the old questions—*why? what?* and *how?*—of theory development have either been put to rest or have undergone major changes. We no longer debate the necessity of unique bodies of theoretical knowledge as bases for either our practice or our existence as a profession. Nor do we question the vital importance of the activities involved in developing such knowledge. We are coming closer to consensus about the appropriate foci of our research; although defined differently in different models, the concepts of people, the environment, nursing, and health are almost universally accepted.[19] Of the original three, only the question of *how* remains.

How to develop nursing theory is being asked in several different ways in today's literature. Fawcett asks us to refine nursing's metaparadigm and further develop our "disciplinary matrixes."[20] Others seek the appropriate methods for studying our concerns and ask whether nursing philosophies and nursing research are in "apposition or opposition."[21] And others seek to reconcile the irreducible nature of holistic phenomena with reductionist methods of science.[22]

Dialectics has been suggested as a way to address today's questions because of the potential that is found in its philosophy, its methods of inquiry and exposition, and its process of intellectual reconstruction and in the dialectical relationship that is assumed to exist among each of these aspects. The dialectical constructs of individuation and abstraction, without betraying holistic phenomena, can provide value for partial knowledge. The dialectic merits our study despite problems that are inherent in its nature, that are predictable given its long history and many interpreters, and that are particular to its close connection with political ideologues of both the left and the right. As one dialectical psychologist has stated: "To ignore it almost constitutes an act of irresponsibility on the part of modern social science.[23]

[19] J. Flaskerud and E. Holloran, "Areas of Agreement in Nursing Theory Development," *Advances in Nursing Science,* 3 (1980), pp. 1–7.

[20] Fawcett, "The Metaparadigm of Nursing."

[21] Munhall, "Nursing Philosophy and Nursing Research."

[22] P. Winstead-Fry, "The Scientific Method and Its Impact on Holistic Health," *Advances in Nursing Science,* 2 (1980), pp. 1–9.

[23] J. F. Rychak, *Dialectic: Humanistic Rationale for Behavior and Development* (Basel, Switzerland: S. Karger, 1976), p. ii.

BEING INFORMED: NURSING RESOURCES FOR THE INFORMATION AGE

VIRGINIA HENDERSON, RN, MA
Senior Research Associate Emeritus
Yale University School of Nursing
New Haven, Connecticut

The work that prepares me to discuss finding information or "being informed" begins with a born tendency to question. For purposes of this discussion, however, the work dates from about 1930 when I began teaching a course at Teachers College of Columbia University that introduced graduate nurses to the scientific method of investigation—problem solving, or "research." After defining the problem to be investigated, the next step was searching the literature for reports of similar or related investigations. Nobody had taught me to search the literature so, enlisting the help of librarians, I taught myself to find and use indexes, abstracts, reviews, and other guides, as well as card catalogues. I soon discovered that few graduate nurses had library skills, and many were afraid to let librarians see their ignorance.

I therefore introduced into this elementary research course a unit on library and bibliographical skills, with librarians helping me teach it. Students were required to give evidence of their competence in using the *Index Medicus,* the *Hospital Index,* the *Reader's Guide, Clinical Abstracts* and other sources. An incidental realization for students was that publications of nursing research were rare, and guides to them—or any other aspect of the nursing literature—were virtually nonexistent.

During the forties I taught a course in advanced medical and surgical

79

nursing for graduate nurse students organized around major clinical problems rather than disease diagnoses grouped under anatomical systems. Searching for answers to clinical problems, students found clinical nursing studies particularly rare and published reports almost impossible to find unless the nurse researcher was a second or third author in a study reported by a physician or other established health scientist. The *Index Medicus* searched and indexed only three or four nursing journals in this era, and there was no short cut to the nursing literature as a whole.

After leaving Teachers College I spent the better part of five years lecturing and revising a wide-ranging nursing text. This kept me acutely aware of nursing's need for library guides and the development of every sort of library resource. As a member of ad hoc committees to persuade nursing organizations to assume responsibility along these lines, I began to realize the extent of resistance or indifference to this idea.

I was therefore glad to be asked in 1953 to join Leo W. Simmons of Yale University in making a survey and assessment of nursing research requested by the National Nursing Service Committee. During the next five years, our staff developed the most extensive bibliographic file then in existence on nursing studies. When Leo Simmons left Yale in 1959, I stayed to prepare this bibliography for publication. The result of this project was the *Nursing Studies Index,* a four-volume annotated index to the analytical, historical, and biographical aspects of the nursing literature published in English from 1900 to 1959.[1]

During and since the preparation of this index, I have worked with nurses, librarians, and others to improve library resources for nursing. This paper is an effort to identify the major accomplishments along these lines and the major tasks that demand attention. Time allows mention of only those that seem most significant in each category; inevitably there will be regrettable omissions. The following topics will be discussed: (1) organizations that promote or should promote improvement of resources, (2) facilities, (3) reference sources, and (4) educational programs.

ORGANIZATIONS, AGENCIES, AND INSTITUTIONS

International

The World Health Organization, the International Council of Nurses (ICN), and the International Labor Organization (ILO) have all indirectly or directly participated in developing reference sources or in conducting investigations that provide nurses with needed information; *none,* however, as far as I know, have committees, departments, or divisions committed to the ongoing improvement of information resources

[1] Virginia Henderson, ed., *Nursing Studies Index* (4 vols.; Philadelphia: J. B. Lippincott, 1963–1972). Now available from Gardner Press, New York City.

for nursing. There is also an International Medical Informatics Association with a branch, the European Federation for Medical Informatics.

As president of the ICN, Margrette Kruse made an effort to develop a standing committee on library resources for nursing. During her presidency, the council worked with the ILO on a survey of working conditions for nurses in countries belonging to the council.

Another example of an international effort is Bishop's bibliography of Florence Nightingale's writings financed by the Florence Nightingale International Foundation.[2] It shows the extent and variety of her impressive output, perhaps second to none in extent, particularly as a correspondent. General knowledge of this bibliography might end the frequent reference by nurses to the recentness of nursing research. No one since has effected so many significant changes in health service as did Florence Nightingale. She was persuasive because she based her recommendations on statistical studies. She is called by some the first medical statistician.

As technology develops, and especially as nurses now play an important role in the design and use of computerized health records, international organizations and agencies will almost certainly see the importance of cooperative use of data banks and the creation of forms that facilitate international employment for health personnel and continuity of care for citizens who move from one country to another. Regional bodies will almost certainly set up workshops and other programs to increase the understanding nurses need along these lines, if they have not already done so. And cartels manufacturing computers and their software will develop departments devoted to this end if for no other than purely selfish interest. The director of a visiting nurse agency recently reported on the computerization of the agency's records.[3] The staff spent 60 percent of its time on paperwork before computerization and made 3.7 visits. After computerization the cost of a visit dropped 20 percent and the number increased to 6.2 in an eight-hour block of time. The association's deficit of $220,000 was converted into a $70,000 surplus.

National

The major national *organizations* in the United States (most specifically the American Nurses' Association, the National League for Nursing Education, and the National League for Nursing) have from time to time had standing or ad hoc committees to promote library resources. Due largely, I believe, to the influence of Isabel M. Stewart, an NLNE

[2] William J. Bishop and Sue Goldie, comps., *A Bio-Bibliography of Florence Nightingale* (London: Dawson of Pall Mall for the International Council of Nursing, 1962).

[3] National Institute of Health, *Second National Conference: Computer Technology and Nursing*, NIH Publ. No. 84-2623 (Washington, D.C.: U.S. Government Printing Office, 1984).

committee prepared guides on the nature, scope, management, and use of libraries and promoted attention to them in creditialing procedures— attention that is still inadequate.

During World War II, the national nursing organizations operated a Nursing Information Bureau in cooperation with the U.S. Public Health Service. This cooperation has continued in the form of an annual statistical volume, *Facts About Nursing*, which is a uniquely valuable service.

Unlike the Canadian Nurses' Association, the Japanese Nursing Association and the Japanese Nursing Publishing Company, and the Royal College of Nursing, the ANA does *not* provide its membership or the public with a national nursing library and its related services. In a paper presented at the 1984 ANA convention, Mussallem gave a long list of the services emanating from the library of the Canadian Nurses' Association.[4] The library of the Royal College of Nursing, at its headquarters on Cavendish Square in London, is accessible even to the general public when it needs information on nursing. This is, I believe, also true of the Japanese Nursing Association's library at its headquarters in Tokyo. However, the most notable service of the Japanese Nursing Association and its publishing company is the number of books and journal articles on nursing published in other languages that it translates into Japanese.

The International Nursing Foundation of Japan has provided an international resource, or library tool, in its volume, *Nursing in the World*.[5] It is a brief "facts on nursing" for the countries belonging to the ICN. Characteristically, this volume is published in both Japanese and English, as is the Japanese Nursing Association's newsletter. Incidentally, the Japanese translate *many* foreign texts and journal articles; we rarely do. In fact, we rarely cite foreign sources, even those written in English.

The national library associations, particularly the Medical Library Association, through its Nursing and Allied Health Resources Section, has promoted the development of library resources for nursing. This is also true of the American Hospital Association and the Catholic Hospital Association.

Of the national *institutions*, the National Library of Medicine is by far the most important. Developed from the Surgeon General's Library, its primary focus has, of course, been medicine. However, General Cummings, its founder, was said in his day to have had the largest nursing collection to be found in this country. Its present organizational structure and the two buildings in Bethesda are designed to serve all health

[4] Helen K. Mussalem, "The Canadian Nurses' Association Library: A National Library Approach." Paper presented at the American Nurses' Association Convention, New Orleans, Louisiana, June 26, 1984.

[5] *Nursing in the World* (Tokyo, Japan: International Nursing Foundation of Japan, 1977).

professionals impartially. Nurses have been members of its board of directors and nurses are employed on its staff. More will be said later about
the nature of its involvement with nursing.

I have left for last a discussion of the two bodies that I believe have
the greatest influence on information sources for American nurses today.
I will discuss first the influence of the American Journal of Nursing Company. It officers can claim that its entire program is committed to the
end of informing. The company has been represented on the committees
of national nursing organizations that have focused on library resources.
The AJN company has developed and operates an outstanding nursing
library. Besides the publication of major American nursing journals,
the company's signal contribution is the publication, in collaboration
with the National Library of Medicine, of the *International Nursing Index*—a
worldwide guide to nursing journals and serial publications. More will
be said about indexes later, but I would like to emphasize the great importance of this publication.

The last national agency is the Interagency Council on Library
Resources for Nursing. As far as I know, it is a unique body with an
unlimited potential for promoting outstanding library resources for the
nursing occupation. The council had its origins in 1959, when Florence
Wald and I were planning the *Nursing Studies Index*. I proposed an advisory committee made up of indexing experts and representatives of
organizations and agencies preparing or promoting guides to the nursing
literature. Florence Wald wisely suggested two committees: one advisory,
composed of experts; the other coordinating, composed of representatives
of organizations, agencies, and institutions that did or might collaborate
in preparing or promoting library resources for nursing.

Both committees were set up. The coordinating committee consisted
of representatives of about a dozen organizations, agencies, and institutions. Meeting at the American Journal of Nursing Company, we almost
immediately constituted ourselves the Interagency Council on Library
Resources for Nursing—an advisory body, without budget. The membership of this council now includes representatives of 27 U.S. nursing or
library and nursing organizations, institutions, and agencies and a
representative of the Canadian Nurses' Association.[6]

---

[6] These agencies are the American Academy of Nursing; American Association of Colleges of Nurs-
ing; American Association for History of Nursing; American Dental Association; American
Hospital Association; American Journal of Nursing Company; American Library Association;
American Medical Association; American Nurses' Association; California Council on Library
Resources/Nursing; Canadian Nurses' Association; Catholic Health Association of the United
States; CINAHL Corporation; Health Sciences Library Association of New Jersey; Medical
Library Association; Mid-Atlantic Regional Archives Conference; National Associaton for Prac-
tical Nurses Education and Service; National Federal of Licensed Practical Nurses; National
League for Nursing; National Library of Medicine; National Student Nurses' Association; New
England Regional Council on Library Resources for Nursing; New England Regional Medical
Library, Nursing Resources Library; New York State Nurses' Association; Nursing Archives,
Mugar Library, Boston University; Sigma Theta Tau; Society for Nursing History; U.S. Public
Health Service, Nursing Division.

We in nursing are fortunate in having a national body of so many able and interested persons who meet for one day biannually to discuss nursing information needs and who work in various ways to meet them. Although I believe the council is uniquely helpful to nursing in this country, its usefulness depends on the extent to which member agencies accept and implement its recommendations.

Regional and State

A New England Council on Library Resources for Nursing has been functioning for several decades, and a California Council on Library Resources for Nursing, recently established, has a comparable structure and function. Largely through the imagination, knowledge, and energy of Mary Pekarsky, nursing librarian at Boston College School of Nursing, and Mary Ann Garrigan, nurse archivist at Boston University School of Nursing, the New England council meetings have been well attended and have stimulated increased awareness among nurses and librarians of the regional resources.

The New York State Nurses' Association at its headquarters in Guilderland has a fine library offering a variety of services to the headquarters staff and to the state membership. If this outstanding achievement was duplicated by all state associations, it would materially affect the development of nursing in this country.

The Pennsylvania League for Nursing has promoted the development of a nursing museum at the Pennsylvania Hospital in Philadelphia. This too might be a model for other states that believe a knowledge of the past furthers understanding of the present.

Most important is the Regional Medical Library Network covering the United States. This is composed of 125 "resource libraries" at medical schools and 2,000 "basic units" (mostly at hospitals) that are served by the National Library of Medicine. The National Library of Medicine has designated a certain number of them as regional health science libraries. Through them, millions of interlibrary loans are made yearly. The Countway Library in Boston is the regional health science library for New England. Because its nursing collection is limited, it uses Boston College's nursing collection as a backup. All health workers and, in fact, the public should know that a regional health science library, partially supported by tax funds, serves the area where they live. Theoretically, these libraries make available to all citizens the National Library of Medicine's computer-based Medical Literature Analysis and Retrieval System (MEDLARS). Actually, the National Library of Medicine offers this as a worldwide service, making available 20 data bases (of which MEDLINE is the best known). MEDLARS is a guide to publications in about 3,000 journals.

Local

Universities, particularly those offering programs for nurses, are promoting information resources for nursing in the United States. Most if not all nursing programs include research courses, and they demand of students the use of library sources and at least rudimentary library and bibliographic skills.

Some university libraries, in collaboration with nursing faculties, have made outstanding contributions. For example, the Mugar Library at Boston University, under the joint leadership of Arthur Gotlieb and Mary Ann Garrigan, has developed a nursing archive that includes the archival material of the American Nurses' Association. (Similar materials from the American Medical Association, the American Dental Association, or the American Hospital Association are found at their headquarters libraries.) Teachers College of Columbia University houses in its library the Adelaide M. Nutting Historical Collection. The University of Missouri makes its nursing collection available to the ANA staff in Kansas City. (This staff does not include a librarian, nor does the center provide substantial library resources.)

Boston College has developed a nursing collection of such excellence that it might serve as a model for health science libraries throughout this country. Mention has already been made of its regional library services.

Hospitals provide libraries that vary greatly in value, but some, particularly those that have combined their medical and nursing holdings, have outstanding resources. The Glendale (California) Adventists Medical Center is an example. Since 1966 it as prepared and published the *Cumulative Index to Nursing Literature,* which is a guide to English language nursing journals, selected journals in allied health, and health science librarianship. It is now computerized, and this data base is available for on-line searching.

This list of local organizations, institutions, and agencies that have made some special contribution to nursing library resources is far from exhaustive, but it provides an introduction to existing resources.

FACILITIES

We tend to call information centers "libraries" and those who help the public use them "librarians." If nursing is to live up to its potential, it must recognize the range of facilities, sources, and services that help us to be informed. Facilities include conventional libraries, resource centers, research centers, computer centers with related data banks, repositories, museums, and archives. Established and affluent professions have developed all of these, and this is by no means an exhaustive list. Many kinds of experts other than librarians are required to staff them.

In this information age, major intellectual tasks are rarely attempted without using computers, because their electronic manipulation of figures or other symbols is so much more rapid than manual manipulation. Nurses, like all other workers, must learn to use modern devices employed in communication or information centers to capitalize on electronic manipulation of data. Those of us who come from diploma programs must learn to be as much at home in large modern facilities as in the small nursing libraries or reading rooms to which we were accustomed as students. Some large libraries are teaching their users to operate computer terminals that request library searches and to be familiar with all the guides to printed and audiovisual sources.

Effective research is built on a knowledge of reported, related research. Grant requests and reports of studies by nurses often fail to include evidence of this knowledge. Nursing practice and teaching, in their scientific aspects, are equally dependent on the effective use of related publications.

Besides information centers that may or may not include historical materials, repositories are essential for the preservation and redistribution of materials not thought to be of immediate use to working libraries. Many libraries are almost useless to students who attempt a long-range study of a subject. I have heard librarians not concerned with a historical approach say, "We discard anything that is more than ten years old." Priceless publications belonging to older nurses are, on their death, destroyed by relatives because the nursing profession has not developed or advertised state or national repositories. The same observation might be made about museums and archives. The University of Missouri School of Nursing Library does have a repository, and other states may as well, but there is not general awareness of them.

REFERENCE SOURCES

Reference sources are library "tools" or guides to information. The Interagency Council on Library Resources for Nursing publishes in *Nursing Outlook* a biennial list of "Reference Sources for Nursing." Resources are arranged in alphabetical order under 16 headings. The following is a slightly modified version of the most recent list.[7]

1. Abstract Journals
2. Audiovisuals (guides to)
3. Bibliographies and Book Lists
4. Computerized Bibliographic Data Bases
5. Dictionaries and Word Books
6. Directories (of nurses and others)

[7] Interagency Council on Library Resources for Nursing, "Reference Sources for Nursing, *Nursing Outlook,* 32 (September-October 1984), pp. 273–277.

7. Directories of Educational Programs
8. Glossaries
9. Histories
10. Indexes
11. Legal Guides
12. Library Administration and Organization Guides
13. Periodical Listings
14. Research and Statistical Sources
15. Research Grants (guides to)
16. Research Reports and Lists

Card catalogues are so well known and standarized that they are not mentioned in this list. They vary greatly in usefulness, however, and may be guides to audiovisual materials as well as books and pamphlets.

A review of the reference sources in this list shows recent gains, but also some obvious failures on the part of nursing to develop adequate reference sources. The most conspicuous accomplishment is publication of indexes to the nursing literature. (The *International Nursing Index* is a companion to the *Index Medicus* and the *Dental Index*.) A conspicuous lack is a directory of nurses (except for those in the U.S. holding doctoral degrees and those who are certified).

Dr. Bayne-Jones, former dean of the Yale Medical School, has said that with the publication of indexes to the nursing literature, the profession "came of age." This is an indication of the importance some people attach to the development and use of guides to the literature. I think the value of practicing nurses to patients depends upon their ability to use the literature, just as the value of educators to students depends upon this ability. Money, time, and effort will continue to be wasted on nursing research until nurse researchers find reports of related research and build on this information. Improvement in nursing practice depends as much on nurses acquiring the habit of finding and applying research in related fields as on conducting studies themselves.

EDUCATIONAL PROGRAMS

There have been, of course, nurse educators who have realized the importance of helping nursing students to acquire working habits that characterize scholarship—but only too few. Workshops on writing are an encouraging recent development. Research courses, which are now a part of most if not all collegiate curricula in this country, demand improved library resources and the rudimentary treatment of bibliographic skills.

However, the programs of international, national, and state conferences, conventions and other meetings rarely include the topics discussed in this paper. In 1969 I reviewed the records of all the ICN Congresses and found only one such session. It was a discussion of textbooks in the late twenties, apparently arranged by Isabel M. Stewart. The Interagency Council on Library Resources for Nursing sponsored a program and an exhibit at the 1969 ICN Congress in Montreal. Neither was mentioned in the published report of the congress. The ICLRN sponsors programs and exhibits at ANA and NLN Conventions, but they are never plenary sessions and they are often poorly attended.

During my long association with nursing education, I have found only one school of nursing requiring all students to demonstrate ability in the use of information sources. This was the diploma program of the Victoria Hospital School of Nursing in London, Ontario, Canada. A semester course was taught around an excellent workbook, with special problems assigned or chosen by students. A librarian participated in the teaching.

With the "publication explosion" and the rapid development of computerized methods, most if not all of us will need instruction, for "self-help" will be the scholar's best hope. It is doubtful whether information centers can afford a sufficiently large staff to give users the service they now need. Some libraries already allow users to operate terminals on which they request literature searches.

Technology comes easier to the young than the old. Nursing students, young and old (like students of law, history, or medicine), would profit by a course of instruction in the techniques of finding information. Exemption examinations could be used to protect the sophisticates among both faculties and student bodies.

SUMMARY

An attempt has been made to suggest the organizations, facilities, reference sources, and educational programs that nursing might develop or use more effectively in helping nurses to be informed. International, national, state, and local organizations, agencies, and institutions need committees or other groups devoted to this objective. Conventional libraries are now accepted as essential to the operation of schools for all health care providers, but nursing students and practicing nurses everywhere should have access to health science information centers that provide a wide range of books, journals, audiovisual materials, data banks, and computer programs. Nursing organizations in this country have not provided their members with all the services they need, but universities have, in certain cases, helped to supply the needed facilities and services.

Educational programs for nurses and student nurses that would give them confidence in the use of facilities, sources, and services are sadly lacking, particularly in the use of computerized data. Recommendations include appointing librarians and other experts to nursing faculties and to the staffs of all agencies that seek full membership in the information age.

BIBLIOGRAPHY

American Nurses' Association. *Directory of Certified Nurses*. Kansas City, Mo.: ANA, 1975.

———. *Directory of Nurses with Doctoral Degrees 1984*. Kansas City, Mo.: ANA, 1984.

———. *Facts About Nursing 82-83*. Kansas City, Mo.: ANA, 1984.

American Nurses' Foundation. *International Directory of Nurses with Doctoral Degrees*. Kansas City, Mo.: ANF.

Bishop, William J. "Florence Nightingale's Letters." *American Journal of Nursing*, 57 (May 1957), p. 607.

———, and Sue Goldie, comps. *A Bio-Bibliography of Florence Nightingale*. London: Dawson of Pall Mall for the International Council of Nursing, 1962.

Bolter, J. David. *Tourings Man: Western Culture in the Computer Age*. Chapel Hill: University of North Carolina Press, 1984.

Canadian Nurses' Association. *Index of Canadian Nursing Studies*. Ottawa, Ontario, Canada: CNA, 1973.

Henderson, Virginia, ed. *Nursing Studies Index*, 4 vols. Philadelphia: J. B. Lippincott, 1963-1972.

Interagency Council on Library Resources for Nursing. "Reference Sources for Nursing." *Nursing Outlook*, 32 (September-October 1984), pp. 273-277.

International Labor Organization. *Employment and Condition of Work and Life of Nursing Personnel*. Geneva, Switzerland: ILO, 1976.

International Nursing Foundation of Japan. *Nursing in the World*. Tokyo, Japan: INFJ, 1977.

Kruse, Margrette. "A World of Unity: From Nationalism to Internationalism." *Imprint*, 20 (April 1973), p. 14.

Mussallem, Helen K. "The Canadian Nurses Association Library: A National Library Approach." Paper presented at the American Nurses' Association Convention, New Orleans, Louisana, June 26, 1984.

Naisbitt, John. *Megatrends: Ten New Directions Transforming Our Lives*. New York: Warner Books, 1982.

National Institute of Health. *Second National Conference: Computer Technology and Nursing*. NIH Publication No. 84–2623. Washington, D.C.: U.S. Government Printing Office, 1984.

National League for Nursing. *Doctoral Programs in Nursing, 1984–85*. New York: NLN, 1985.

_____. *NLN Nursing Data Book, 1983–84*. New York: NLN, 1984.

Nutting, M. Adelaide. "Florence Nightingale as a Statistician," *Public Health Nurse*, 19 (May 1927), p. 207.

Simmons, Leo W., and Virginia Henderson. *Nursing Research: A Survey and Assessment*. New York: Appleton-Century-Crofts, 1964.

THE IMPACT OF COMPUTERS ON NURSING

SUSAN J. GROBE, RN, PhD, FAAN
Associate Professor of Nursing
School of Nursing
University of Texas at Austin

The central theme of my remarks about computers and their impact on nursing curricula are captured in two quotations and a short story. They dramatize my thoughts about the effects of technology on nursing and the health care professions.

The first quotation is about nursing science: "Computers are capable of profoundly affecting science by stretching human reason and intuition, much as telescopes and microscopes extended human vision."[1] The second quotation, attributed to Oliver Wendell Holmes, pertains to nursing education and practice: "The mind, once expanded to the dimensions of larger ideas, never returns to its original size." And finally, the short story is about time and the future:

> A young man on the beach in North Carolina in December, 1903 watched Orville and Wilbur Wright begin aviation. His father proclaimed, "Son, you just saw the future...."
>
> Some 80 years later, the son, living in Southern California is awakened from a sound sleep by a sonic boom as the space shuttle lands. His comment, "There's a lot more future coming...."[2]

Thus, my two major themes about technology and nursing are first, that computers are capable of affecting our thinking, our lives, our science, and our profession in ways we cannot yet fully visualize; and second, that the shift to a computer-based technology will stretch us to new limits—while at the same time reminding us constantly that "there's a lot more future coming."

---

[1] A. Oettinger and S. Marks, *Run Computer Run* (Cambridge, Mass.: Harvard University Press, 1969).

[2] R. Gray, "The Future's Arrived," *Infoworld* (July 9, 1984), p. 7.

THE PRESENT AND THE FUTURE

How do we distinguish between what is the present and what is the future? Some examples can help. Consider the time when:

- Commencement means a degree and a permanent access number to a specialized data base—that is, access to a constantly changing data base that contains all known nursing knowledge and the most recently published health care research.

- Employment criteria for differing types of nursing positions categorize them as "thinking" and "nonthinking" positions.

- Large organizations such as universities, corporations, health agencies, and state and federal governmental bodies have telecommunication capabilities that preclude any necessity for physical proximity; learners in those institutions no longer write on paper with pencils, but use word processing almost exclusively and communicate with professors via electronic networks.

- Learners use computer simulations to solve substantial, realistic problems using massive amounts of real-world data; students of the sciences and professions learn by discovery rather than by notetaking; and learning to solve problems, thought, and reasoning take precedence over the struggle to accumulate information.

- Organizational structures are designed to include research and development in a collaborative scientific inquiry model that blends scholars and practitioners in basic research processes.

- Invisible colleges and scholars with similar inquiries are tied together with global communication networks, irrespective of national and organizational boundaries.

- Education is truly an introduction to scholarly thinking and continuing education for life.

Although for some, these examples may seem futuristic, in fact, these situations represent the present in many arenas of today's society. Based on our knowledge of what currently exists, however, how can we meet the challenges that computer technology poses for nursing and nursing education? Among the questions to be answered are: What needs to be learned? What do we select to teach? How do we organize it? What are our goals?

Specifically, does nursing focus on the *computer as a tool* to be mastered, or does it focus on the *nature of computing* as an important topic and issue for nursing? Do we prepare the "user" who merely uses the latest tool as it is provided, the "thinking user" who commands the tool for practice purposes, or the "knowledgeable user" who masters the tool and uses it creatively for the improvement of nursing science and nursing practice? Are our goals focused on detailing the present or projecting the future? How are professional nurses prepared for the constancy of change associated with the uncertainty of the technological future? These are nursing's challenges.

Prior to discussing the important choices about how technology can be incorporated into nursing curricula, I will examine some general effects of computer technology in four areas: the professions, organizations, patterns of communication, and scientific inquiry. This will help set the context for understanding what nursing's curricular alternatives are and how our choices might be made. Then I will discuss the implications of changes in each of these areas for nursing practice and curricula.

IMPACT OF COMPUTER TECHNOLOGY

Professions

The effects of the computer on individuals' personal as well as professional lives are called to our attention constantly by the mass media, which tells us that an educated individual must possess that nebulous attribute known as computer literacy, and that computer illiteracy condemns one to life on the margin of the coming information society. Particularly distressing is the parallel drawn with literacy by the careless use of the term, *computer literacy*.

As others have stated, we teach reading and writing skills so that learners can absorb the facts of civilization and can also encounter the very structure of style, thought, and imagination. Thus, true literacy for professionals is achieved when a professional thinks better and thinks differently using the information he or she has read. Literacy for professionals, then, is more than possession of reading and writing skills. It is much more than recognizing a book and its words. Professional individuals are not literate unless they can deal with the content of books—that is, the literature—rather than just the mechanics of its form.

In a similar sense, computer literacy for professionals is more than just knowing how computers operate and how to use certain software. Computer literacy is best defined as having enough contact with the technology and skill with computing activities to reach the level of fluency and understanding of its use for professional purposes. Computer literacy for professionals is the ability to use the machine and the information it provides to think better—a natural use for professional nursing practice and nursing science. Professional nurses must be both "thinking" and "knowledgeable" users of technology—more than is implied in the media definition of computer literacy.

Another aspect of computers' use is also important for health care professionals. Smith categorizes jobs in our new information age into two types: the "thinking" and "nonthinking." "Those who succeed in the work force will be those who have learned to learn. The unthinking jobs will be done by machine."[3] Smith's evidence is quite convincing. Consider two relevant examples. One engineering technician with a computer can do in one day tasks that one month ago took a draftsman three weeks to complete. One statistician with a computer can perform in one morning calculations that only recently took a statistician several days. If the repetitive and routine tasks of measuring, drawing, and calculating associated with engineering and statistics can be done efficiently by technicians using the computers, the professional architect is free to formulate designs to be implemented, and the professional researcher is free to designate the statistics to be analyzed. Thus, computers have become essential professional efficiency tools.

These examples easily extend to nursing, especially to the realm of planning and documenting patient care. Consider the potential impact of freeing the nurse from the drudgery of routine and repetitive clerical tasks and freeing the professional's mind to attend to the larger ideas of nursing science. The computer can be an efficient tool, useful for nursing science.

Organizations

Computers also affect professionals in their organizational settings, including nurses in complex health care organizations. Preliminary research by Harriman suggests that computers affect patterns of communication within organizations.[4] Computer technology has freed many organizations of the physical constraints necessitating centralized organizational structures. Greater flexibility in use and scheduling of employees, wider dispersion of employees, and rewards based on productive output rather than on time input, are but a few effects. Another unanticipated effect has been an increase in routinization and standardization of many organizational procedures. Administrators in computerized organizations demonstrate an increased capacity to supervise both employees and the ongoing processes of an organization using sophisticated data base audits.

Patterns of Communication

Czajowski reports research describing the effects of computer technology on social and professional interactions and communication

[3] C. E. Smith, "Education, the Workplace and High Technology," *National Forum*, 64, No. 2 (1984), p. 45.

[4] A. Harriman, "The Rise and Fall of the Third Wave," *National Forum*, 64 (Summer 1984), pp. 20–30.

patterns in organizations.[5] Computer networks have increased access to information within organizations, while reducing the accompanying social information, such as eye contact, tone of voice, and nonverbal gestures. Resulting communications via computer networks are more direct, frank, revealing, and uninhibited. In effect, messages sent and received via electronic networks are longer and stronger.

Czajowski also notes that decisions made via electronic networks in organizations are judged to be "more extreme" and "less influenced" by authority figures. Thus, decision making via electronic networks seems to be more equally shared among all participants. An interesting side effect of the "electronic suggestion box" has been these networks' gradual metamorphosis into employee "gripe networks." Several of these networks have been discontinued in organizations because of their detrimental effects on employee morale. These examples of altered communication patterns apply especially to the patterns of communication among nurses and other health care providers.

Scientific Inquiry

Finally, computers are affecting our views of science and the ways we explore, discover, organize, and disseminate information. Computer technology allows scientists to aggregate data, instances, and examples and to analyze them for meaning. This analysis and synthesis requires that human scientists enter Peterson's world of symbolics in human experience, in which humans, noting repetitious instances, are motivated to exchange this boring repetition for single abstract insights or to generate what some theorists call the "aha!" of science.[6]

Computers allow scientists to discover patterns, regularities, and rules in nature and humanity. For example, Wolfram describes how computer simulation has made it practical to consider many new kinds of models for physical, mathematical, and natural phenomena:

> Physical objects and mathematical structures can be represented as numbers and symbols. . .and a program can be written to manipulate them according to the algorithms. When the computer program is executed, it causes the numbers and symbols to be modified in the way specified by the scientific laws. . . [and] thereby allows the consequences of the laws to be deduced. . . .Computation thus extends the realm of experimental science: It allows experiments to be performed in a hypothetical universe."[7]

[5] A. Czajowski and S. Kiesler, "Computer Mediated Communication," *National Forum*, 64 (Summer 1984), pp. 31-34.

[6] N. Peterson, "Designing a Simulated Laboratory," *Byte*, 9, No. 6 (1984), pp. 287-296.

[7] S. Wolfram, "Computer Software in Science and Mathematics," *Scientific American*, 251, No. 3 (1984), p. 188.

This concept applies to the study of social behaviors and nursing science. The complexity of what can be modeled is increasing. As Wolfram states:

> Computation is making possible the study of phenomena far more complex than ones that could previously be considered, and it is changing the direction and emphasis of many fields of science. Perhaps most significant, it is introducing a new way of thinking in science. . . . Scientific laws are now thought of as algorithms. New aspects of natural phenomena have been made accessible to investigation.[8]

Some of these newly accessible natural phenomena are likely to affect the realm of health care and nursing.

Computers also have implications for scientific research when they serve as controllers for machines and processes in the workaday world. Use of computer controllers for air traffic, nuclear power plants, telephone networks, and spacecraft guidance are but a few examples. The model of the process governs the computer. In health care, research on the use of controllers for specific complex tasks is well underway. Intravenous drug administration and complex physiological monitoring and alert systems are but a few of the many examples. The complex knowledge needed for designing and advancing such technology is of inestimable value in health care situations and settings. Health care is benefitting now from many innovations of the National Aeronautics and Space Administration (NASA).

Computer technology also allows scientists to extend the world of information beyond the hierarchically structured boundaries of formal reasoning into problem solving, a closely guarded realm of the various professions. The medical profession calls these programs ''medical consultation systems.'' Although success has not yet been achieved in finding computer solutions to general problems using less formal rules of thumb, there have been successful artificial intelligence programs in limited and special knowledge domains close to the health professions. MYCIN, DENDRAL, ONCOCIN, and AI-RHEUM are but a few of these programs in medicine.[9] Nursing has not yet developed artificial intelligence programs.

A profession's power rests with the expert practitioner's use of knowledge and rules of knowledge. However, development of computer software for intelligent systems has illustrated that much of a professional's knowledge is intuitive and context bound and is not easily converted to formal rules.[10] This has implications for nursing, where the

---

[8] *Ibid.*

[9] S. J. Grobe, *Computer Primer and Resource Guide for Nurses* (Philadelphia: J. B. Lippincott Co., 1984).

[10] T. Alexander, ''Why Computers Can't Outthink the Experts,'' *Fortune,* 110 (August 20, 1984), pp. 105–118.

domain is large and the language quite imprecise. "Many early artificial intelligence programs depended heavily on formal reasoning methods . . . and, for formal reasoning to work as the sole source of power in a program . . . the problem must be small."[11]

IMPLICATIONS FOR NURSING AND CURRICULA

What do these notions about the impact of computer technology mean for the future of nursing and for nursing curricula? I will examine a few of these generalizations.

Professional Nurses

The first notion described was that of computer literacy for professionals. Can we define it for nursing? What is "enough contact" with computers to reach a level of fluency and understanding? Remember, computer literacy for professionals is the ability to use the machine and its information to think better—in this case, about science and about nursing.

Therefore, computer literacy for nurses is more than just knowing the use of software, word processing capability, use of data-base management, use of research and statistics, or design of programming and software. Rather, it is actually using the technology and its various software programs to begin asking questions and gathering evidence for solving problems in nursing practice, education, research, and administration. Computer literacy implies well-prepared professionals who are concerned with technology and its uses as well as the ethical and legal issues inherent in its use in health care.

In this regard, nursing curricula must prepare professional nurses as thinking users. This requires that learners balance "what is" with "what could be." On the one hand, we must educate students about the present uses of computers in nursing practice, education, administration, and research. On the other hand, we must help them consider the potential computers have for health care and the profession. The latter challenge includes preparing thinking and knowledgeable nurses who can participate fully in seeing that this potential is achieved.

Also bearing on curricular considerations is the question of whether there are "thinking" and "nonthinking" tasks in nursing. What repetitive tasks and routine jobs can be done safely by machine? And what tasks will be reserved for those who have learned to learn? Using nursing record keeping as an example, it is fairly easy to sort out the routine from the nonroutine tasks of record keeping. A nurse must adjust the standard care plan and individualize it for the particular patient. Machines can automatically record the care plan and the regularly monitored vital signs

---

[11] D. B. Lenat, "Computer Software for Intelligent Systems," *Scientific American*, 251, No. 3 (1984), pp. 204–213.

and laboratory results. However, if an alert sounds, indicating impending metabolic acidosis, for example, a thinking nurse must validate the readings, adjust the IV flow and the respirator settings, and reset the alert alarm for subsequent readings. The automated record-keeping system can record the changes and reinitialize (reset) the system's remaining elements. The "thinking" professional nurse's understanding of what adjustments must be made for the patient would probably be derived from a query of the patient's electronic data base.

A "knowledgeable" nurse might go even further in using technology for nursing science purposes. The knowledgeable nurse might select the patient's situational parameters and make additional queries to determine which of several key interacting variables could be used to predict successful nursing interventions in similar patient situations. For example, what prognosis could be expected for this patient or for patients like him or her? What are the typical nursing problems to anticipate? What are the most likely and most successful interventions for similar patients with similar situational variables?

A carefully designed data base, with data useful for nursing, can provide this wealth of experiential knowledge for advancing nursing science. However, the capability to access the information and use it effectively and successfully is within the professional nurse's realm only if the knowledgeable nurse can adequately use the computer as a tool to define, access, and use the information for nursing science purposes.

Therefore, curricula for preparing thinking and knowledgeable nurses must include information to help nurses become informed and skillful users of computer technology. Nurses must know about computer systems, their design, their implementation, and their evaluation. With such knowledge, thinking and knowledgeable professional nurses can help vendors with the design and evaluation of technological systems that are truly useful for nursing practice and nursing science.

Communication and Health Care Organizations

The ideas discussed regarding electronic communication and the impact of computer technology organizations raise many questions for nursing and nursing curricula. If the organizational patterns of hospitals and health care settings remain constant, what can nurses anticipate? And if patterns of care provision change, how can nursing respond? Will increased electronic communication with other health care providers allow more equal input into patient care decisions? Will decentralized delivery of patient care and increased reliance on electronic communication networks increase professional nursing's responsibility for patient follow-up activities? Will more routinized and standardized care protocols follow? Will increased levels of responsibility associated with increased participation in decision making about care be accompanied by more audit and supervisory control? Or, will nurses lose their central place as the mediator (not just communicator) of patient information?

If the large, centralized health care agencies become decentralized, where and how will the professional nurse continue to practice? And in what capacity? As an employee of an agency, or as a professional practitioner? What are the parameters of professional practice? How will it be defined, and by whom? What is its future? What resources are available for health care services, and will current reimbursement practices dictate what nursing practice is? What will changing patterns of reimbursement and organization, spurred on by technological change, mean for nursing? What are the implications for nursing curricula?

Rapid electronic communication and organizational changes associated with technology have helped to emphasize the necessity for including and examining closely in nursing curricula the nature of change and ways for professionals to continually keep up-to-date in order to deal with it. Awareness of the false solidity of knowledge—its constantly changing nature—must be emphasized as a stark reality for lifetime professional practice. Recognition of the timeliness of information and the necessity of remaining up-to-date are equally as important in nursing curricula as the accumulation of the knowledge base of scientific facts.

As Henderson has so ably stated, "If you can't access the best and most timely information and knowledge, then you can't practice quality nursing care."[12] Evaluative studies on health care computing systems support Henderson's assertion. As the quality of information available for care increases, so does the quality of care possible. Our curricula and continuing education programs must ensure that professional nurses understand the importance of the relationship between information and quality care. Further, nurses must learn how to use the electronic tools to communicate and to access the most recent scientific knowledge and information.

Nursing Science

Just as scientists' ways of exploring knowledge using computers continue to expand, so too will nurses' capabilities. As we know, computers allow us to store data, to aggregate data, and to analyze data in order to abstract meaning from them. Existing data are a fruitful resource for nurses in formulating meaningful insights about individuals' health responses, healthful life patterns, and nursing interventions. The science of nursing, health, and health care delivery has so many unasked and unanswered questions. Many of the answers reside in large electronic data bases or in electronic patient records.

---

[12] V. Henderson, "Nursing and the New Technology," presentation at the National League for Nursing First National Conference on Nursing Education, Philadelphia, Pennsylvania, December 1984.

Learning to use electronic tools to examine literature and research data bases is thus an essential skill for professional nurses. Its principles and its practice should be included in nursing curricula and continuing education programs. Knowledgeable nurses must understand the necessity for balancing the traditional literature search strategies with electronic computer search strategies for staying professionally up-to-date.[13] And nurse scientists must be precise and comprehensive in titling their works to ensure that searches of the data base provide access to the desired information. Professional nurses must think of themselves as scientists with an obligation to advance nursing knowledge and nursing theory.

CONCLUSIONS

Nursing curricula must include experiences that ensure preparation of nurses as skillful users of technology. The desirable level of preparation dictates that curricula and continuing education programs contain "hands-on" learning experiences to prepare thinking and knowledgeable nurses. We must prepare nurses who know how to use these tools for scientific inquiry about practice and for staying current with the knowledge and information essential for quality nursing practice.

Faculty need to be prepared for incorporating technology within nursing curricula. An acute need exists to challenge faculty to develop and maintain a tolerance for change, an appetite for continued learning, and a sincere effort to stay abreast of the technological crest—capacities so essential for our profession's effort. Nursing cannot let it be said that we failed, that we did not recognize the opportunity to capture computer technology and use it to assist us in examining nursing, developing nursing science, and advancing the nursing profession.

[13] R. Fox and M. Ventura, "Efficiency of Automated Literature Search Mechanisms," *Nursing Research*, 34, No. 3 (1984), pp. 204–213.

STATE-OF-THE-ART TECHNOLOGY: COMPUTERS AND CURRICULUM

GARY D. HALES, PhD
Editor-in-Chief, *Computers in Nursing*
Software Acquisition and Development Director
J. B. Lippincott Company
Houston, Texas

One major obstacle to implementing computer technology in nursing education is that one must be able to communicate with the experts in this area; to do that, one must speak the jargon. For this reason, terms that may be unfamiliar or used in special ways are defined throughout this article.

Currently, the situation in development of hardware and software is somewhat chaotic. Any number of promising companies have declared bankruptcy and have either reorganized or left the marketplace altogether. These conditions reflect the volatile nature of this industry; those companies with the vision to correctly predict the most needed products and the technological advances to build these products are going to succeed. This "shakeout" of companies, long predicted and often falsely reported, has resulted in a settling of the computer industry. For example, the Fall 1984 COMDEX trade show—the major industry showcase—was notable for its lack of explosive surprises and secret projects. Instead, the sessions had a staid, business-oriented atmosphere. Those companies that had made correct decisions were learning how to occupy their niches more comfortably and expand cautiously. Whereas the Fall 1983 COMDEX had been exciting and dynamic, one left the 1984 show somewhat bored but feeling that the computer industry had begun to come out of the doldrums.

NEW DEVELOPMENTS IN TECHNOLOGY

Despite the few surprises at the meeting, developments in product areas suggested significant trends in software and hardware. One of these areas was telecommunications. The advances in telecommunications were

101

focused primarily on high-speed modems (the 2,400 baud variety), local area network systems (LANS) and micro-to-mainframe communications.[1] One impact of these developments on nursing education will be an opportunity to develop nontraditional classrooms and expand the chances for continuing education. Instead of having students or faculty physically present for lectures or workshops, it will become increasingly popular to gather people together over telephone lines for electronic conferences. It is costly to send participants to continuing education sessions, but the need for such activities will continue to grow rather than diminish. If one makes effective use of telecommunications, however, personnel in need of continuing education can have access to instructors and course material without leaving the environs of their office. This not only reduces costs but also eliminates travel time.

The new local area network systems and software can also be considered as advances in telecommunications because they allow a number of microcomputers to be linked together using modems, cables, or both. Networks to be introduced in the next two years will be reasonable in cost and much easier to install and will be accompanied by software that allows sharing of peripherals and efficient use of archival storage devices.[2] This is not to state that mainframe computers will become a thing of the past.

---

[1] *Modems (modulator-demodulator):* A device that converts computer output to audio signals, can transmit these signals over telephone lines, and can decipher such signals from other computers. The modem allows the computer user to make contact with other computers and use large *data bases* (organized collections of data) or communication networks.

Baud: The rate at which characters are sent or received over some type of communications link. Typical baud rates are 300 and 1200, meaning 30 or 120 characters (letters, numbers, etc.) are sent or received per second.

Microcomputer: A small computer system with its own *CPU* (central processing unit—the "brain" that directs the computer's operations), usually designed for one user, and with speed and performance inferior to that of a *minicomputer* (a medium-sized computer) or *mainframe* computer.

Mainframe: A large computer (physically and functionally) accommodating hundreds of users, offering many *languages* (sets of conventions and rules directing programming), capable of handling extensive and lengthy calculations quickly, and possessing many devices for *input* and *output* (getting data into and out of the computer).

[2] *Peripherals:* Devices that are, literally, peripheral to the actual operation and use of the computer. Although the computer can function without peripherals, they are necessary to be able to make use of the products of the computer's labor. Peripherals include card readers, printers, joy sticks or paddles used with games, data storage devices, etc.

Storage devices: Units used to store information when the computer is turned off. The most common storage devices include disks and tapes. *Disks* look something like a record and, using the accompanying *drive,* allow relatively immediate access to any point on the disk. Flexible *floppy disks* are commonly used in microcomputers and have storage capacities of up to one *megabyte*— one million characters (this is now being exceeded). *Hard disk* drives use rigid disks, which spin at a much faster rate, resulting in much faster storage or retrieval, and have storage capacity of five megabytes (five million characters) and up. With *tape,* one can store large amounts of information, but the access is sequential—that is, the tape must be physically moved to the location of the information to permit reading; this is slower than disk access. *Streaming* tape drives use a continuous tape to store large amounts of data quickly.

The micro-to-mainframe connection refers to software and hardware systems designed to make communications between the two types of systems—that is, sharing of data and programs—easy and painless, even for the novice user. New software now being developed will enable the user to conduct statistical analyses on one computer using data stored on another. There will also be increased use of microcomputers in the hospital; all the advantages inherent in distributed processing (using stand-alone work stations to do some of the work normally done by the mainframe computer) will be joined with the large data storage capacity and high-speed processing power of the mainframe computers.

Another significant trend is the development of what might be called ergonomically designed software. Just as ergonomic furniture fits the human contour and complements human physical limitations (such as susceptibility to eye fatigue when viewing computer screens in glaring light), ergonomic software permits the use of programs in more natural ways. Obscure and easily forgotten commands will be replaced by simple to use menus and mnemonic commands that have some easily understood relationship to the results of using the commands.[3] Instead of having to work with one program at a time, the user can "open a window" to a second program on one part of the screen. For example, while in the middle of a word-processing session, the user might choose to leave a note in a colleague's electronic mailbox. Rather than wait until editing of the manuscript is finished and risk forgetting to leave the message, the user can open a window into a mailing program by assigning a small segment of the viewing screen for that program. The user can then leave the message and resume editing the material— material that has remained on the screen the entire time. Software developers are beginning to learn that people do not simply want software, they want software that can be used.

Whereas telecommunications relates to having computers access each other easily, portability means having computers where users can access them whenever they need to. Up to this point, the user has been limited to using the computer where there was an electric source and, usually, all the typical accoutrements of the normal office. Even the so-called portable computers—the lap-top and transportable models—do not really alleviate the need for a computer at home base because of either their incompatibility with computers in the office, the lack of applications software, or the sheer inconvenience of hauling around a 30-pound box.[4] Now, there are lap-top computers with disk drives, 24-line displays, and the all-important factor of IBM compatibility. Thus, nurses can have a computer that will tie into the computers at the office when they make community health visits for data collection and patient education, col-

---

[3] *Menu:* List of possible commands from which to choose desired functions.

[4] *Applications software:* Programs designed for a particular job, such as word processing or spread sheets.

lect data for research, need a traveling office, or wish to extend the time computers are available in a learning center. We are reaching a point where the only distance limitation in the use of microcomputers will be financial resources. Computing is where you need it, not where the electric plug is.

IMPLEMENTING THE TECHNOLOGY

There is no question that great changes are taking place in the classroom at all levels. In the college classroom, computers can be used for, among other things, demonstrations, experiments, teaching statistics, and, of course, teaching students about the computer. Of equal interest, however, and even more important for integrating computers into the curriculum, is the impact on the learning center. The faculty must be heavily involved with the decision to integrate computers into the curriculum, because they will be the ones who will know what software is needed in the classroom. In addition, the faculty can motivate their students to use the computer, thus justifying the time and money that will be required.

The steps in developing a plan to use computers in the learning center involve answering the following questions: *what* you are going to do; to *whom* and with whom you will do it; *where* the installation will take place; and *when* you plan to do it. You should also not neglect the "how" question; that is, how you will pull together all the diverse elements and how you obtain the materials (hardware and software) needed to bring the plan to fruition. The answers to all these questions will be unique to your institution.

What you are going to do means planning the course work to be supplemented or replaced with software. This entails careful consideration of the software available, the frequency with which courses are taught, which courses are required and which are elective, average enrollment, and any other factor that one would normally consider when examining how one part of the curriculum relates to another. Consider the computer as a new faculty member; consider how you would assign this person, with finite skills and experience (available software) to courses in the curriculum.

The "who" question is twofold. First, one must decide who—that is, which students—needs exposure soonest. It may be that you want to start using computers for teaching remedial material that many students need but that faculty are loath to teach. Perhaps you will want to focus on senior students; they may need access to and understanding of computer systems in order to fit smoothly into the normal hospital routine. The second "who" question relates to the people who will be delivering the training or working with the computers. In addition to some administrative and technical personnel, plan to involve faculty members or staff who are already sold on computers. This is not the time to make converts to the cause; those who are reluctant will either adapt or become obsolete.

The question of *where* has actually become much more exciting with the advent of the portable computer described earlier. Now the learning center or computer laboratory can be open all night. If a computer can be checked out overnight or for weekend use, the hours of access can be extended without adding personnel. This also means encouraging use of the computer in nontraditional places, such as collecting data from a patient in the hospital, doing patient education at the bedside, and so forth. With the new machines, you must forget the physical dimensions of the room and think of the computer lab as anywhere that faculty or students may be involved in instruction, patient care, or research.

"When" is a question with one constant and one variable answer. The first answer to this question is always "as soon as possible." The integration of computers into the college curriculum and into the world of work is only going to accelerate. Any school that does not take this into account might as well ask the dinosaurs to move over and make room. That the school should begin, after thoughtful planning, to implement computers as soon as possible is a given, You should, however, give careful thought to the timetable involved. No matter what you are planning, I strongly recommend that you do not plan for more than a three-year period, because the technology is likely to change dramatically in three years. The new trends and the new possibilities will suggest very different applications than one would consider based on the technology available in 1985. By planning for three years and building in periodic opportunities for modification in plans, you will be able to take advantage of the newest software and hardware. You should also know that most computer equipment you buy will be obsolete in three years or less. Obsolete does not mean useless, however; it means that although you can still use the equipment, it does not have the latest developments and will not be able to take advantage of the latest trends in software. Since software is the factor that really makes the computer more than just a paperweight, you should always plan your computer use with one eye on future developments in software.

SELECTING SOFTWARE

Evaluating software is, or at least ought to be, a systematic and orderly process. Software should always be selected before selecting the hardware. If you follow this advice, you will be able to choose the most economical computer system that runs the software you want. If you choose the computer first, you might be forced to accept software that does not fully meet your needs but is the only program available given the computer you have chosen. In order to add some measure of order to the software selection process, I have developed the checklist included in Figure 1. It should be noted that this particular form has not been validated or had reliability established as yet.

While this evaluation form is to be used with any piece of software, I have provided an additional set of questions specific to the purchase of educational software. For specific administrative or business applications (such as word processing, general ledger, or data bases), consult the software reviews in computer publications.

Good educational software—or, for that matter, any software—should be ergonomically designed. That is, the challenge to the student should be learning the material, not mastering the program operation. The documentation (accompanying manuals) for simple programs should be simple too. The only documentation that should be lengthy is that involving a teaching process, since the very concept is difficult or new. A statistics program, for example, might provide descriptions of the statistical techniques to enhance use.

The actions the user is required to perform should be logical and clearly explained on-line. You should not have to accept glitches simply to get software. After you view a few programs, you will quickly learn how to spot elegantly designed software. At that point, you need to pay close attention to content or have a content expert evaluate it for you.

STATE OF THE FUTURE

Just as the technology changes rapidly, so does the terminology associated with that technology. Although a number of terms have already been considered and will remain important in determining your use of computers, still more terms will become essential in the near future.

One of the primary considerations is that computer memory is getting cheaper all the time. What this means to the user is that the programs can be more sophisticated and yet easier to use. Programmers can build in more "help" screens and construct the programs to make their use more logical and consistent. In addition, the programs can do more—for example, word processing and telecommunications in one package—for less money. It is now possible to use some very elegant and broad statistical programs on microcomputers, for instance. Perhaps the best way to appreciate the meaning of more memory is to examine programs that were considered sophisticated even two years ago and look at the newest versions today.

As available RAM continues to increase, the computer user will have many more capabilities in even smaller machines.[5] The greater memory will also allow the developers of programs to build software that will mimic the capabilities of one-on-one instruction even more than current

---

[5] *RAM:* Random access memory; the memory available to the user for workspace and storage of instructions, programs, and data.

software. For example, one of the problems with some current computer-assisted instruction (CAI) software is that it is limited in its capacity to accept string input (in this case, words, phrases, or sentences) as opposed to merely allowing multiple-choice entries. Wouldn't it be nice to have a program that could examine the contents of an open-ended essay type of question? The instructor could have the program search for key phrases indicating grasp of the material.

While on-line memory will continue to get cheaper, there will remain a need for large off-line storage devices. The laser disk will permit one to store gigabytes—billions of characters—on the same medium now used to watch *Superman* or *Raiders of the Lost Ark*. The disk is durable and the storage and retrieval speeds are very fast, incorporating the same random-access capability that distinguishes floppy disks from sequential access tapes. The presentation can be under computer control, so that one can search for and display a particular image very quickly. The fact that this medium may be used to show visual images such as slides has obvious implications for libraries that house visual images that nurses need to consult.

One of the most exciting new trends is the development of cellular telecommunications equipment. Whereas even two years ago mobile phones were expensive and limited in number, the new cellular phones will make the ability to telephone from anywhere available to many more people. Eventually, I expect to see telephones in computers. For example, the small lap-top computer does not need an electric plug to operate; it uses a battery pack. As discussed earlier, this means that computing goes where you need it. The next step is to put telecommunications capability inside this small box. Then you will be able to have the computer, with no wires, cables, or plugs, not only work with you in a rural farm area, but also communicate "through the ether" with another computer located in the heart of New York City. You can use a cellular phone to call New York from that farmhouse now; soon your computer will have the same opportunity.

THE EDUCATIONAL IMPACT

Three of the areas in which the newest technology will have a major impact on education are simulations, continuing education, and authoring.

Simulations. The simulations that will be available with the new technology will go beyond the text-dependent scenarios common today and will routinely incorporate high-quality video and graphics, as well as interaction between the computer and videocassette and videodisk machines. As the computer systems become more sophisticated, simulations will also, involving more than one student and much more realistic situations. Thus, half a dozen individuals might participate in one simulated clinical scene.

Continuing education. There will also be dramatic changes in the whole area of adult learning in general and continuing education in particular, as lessons are delivered via cable television, satellite, and diskette, with extensive interaction between the trainer, whether human or machine, and the learner. It is becoming cost-effective to utilize electronic means to distribute information.

Authoring. Authoring programs are designed to allow the nonprogrammer to use the computer to develop such things as lesson plans for CAI, making lesson development much easier. An authoring system translates plain English commands into a language that the computer can understand. Authoring systems allow the user to develop CAI that is specific to a particular curriculum and environment. There will still be a need, however, for attention to the instructional design. In many cases, there will also be need for a programmer to take the basic skeleton built by the user of the authoring system and add sophisticated graphics or other routines not available in most authoring packages.

All these developments have publishers wondering what to do. One solution is to simply go with the flow and try, often unsuccessfully, to determine where the flow is going. The difficulty in this determination arises from the fact that the flow of technology and innovation often trickles off into dead-end ponds. Many a company has stagnated in such a pond. Companies—at least the less adventurous ones—will, unfortunately, continue to avoid making making things happen and responding to needs. The companies that will be successful will study the trends and attempt to anticipate the needs. The age of the entrepreneur, of the "garage geniuses," will not end, however; as computers continue to proliferate, so will the users. Many of the brightest ideas will come from this user base—ideas that large companies will purchase and promote as small developers cannot. This is what will keep this industry dynamic—the input of bright, creative users.

CONCLUSION

There is wise saying regarding to whom the future belongs. In the case under discussion, the future and those populating it will be the property of the administrators—and, therefore, the schools—that are willing to put away tradition and strike out in new areas. In many cases, these schools will be pioneering; there will be no signposts except the ones they leave behind. Over the last five years, there have been many false starts, but the schools that started the earliest and began looking for unmarked trails are still leading the way. The danger of working with a new technology is that one becomes comfortable in the lead and gets lazy; this results in stagnation and loss of leadership. If you have begun using computers and the accompanying technology in the curriculum, push your people and resources to the limit daily. If you have not yet started, learn from the mistakes of your compatriots and begin today.

Figure 1. Software Evaluation Checklist*

Directions: The four-point scale ranges from 1 (agree very much) to 4 (disagree very much). For questions that are not relevant to your needs, circle N/A (not applicable); but please read each item carefully, as it may suggest some element that you have overlooked.

Title of program: _____

Type of program: _____

Description of the program, i.e., what is it supposed to do?:_____

_____

_____

Language written in: _____ Price: _____

Hardware needed:_____

Author(s): _____ Source or Publisher: _____

Target audience: _____

Usage history: _____

General Evaluation Questions

Use

1. Does the software address your needs?   1 2 3 4 N/A

2. Does the software make full use of the computer's capabilities? You do not want to waste your money on something that could be done simpler, better, or cheaper using print media or video.   1 2 3 4 N/A

3. Is the scope of the program reasonable?   1 2 3 4 N/A

4. Are directions unambiguous?   1 2 3 4 N/A

5. Is the program easy to operate? This may mean menu driven or with use of function keys a la IBM.   1 2 3 4 N/A

6. Is the program flow logical?   1 2 3 4 N/A

7. Is the package free of programming errors?   1 2 3 4 N/A

8. Can the user request help at any time?   1 2 3 4 N/A

9. Can the user exit the program and save work (if desired) at any point?   1 2 3 4 N/A

---

10. Does the program "lock out" inappropriate key presses?   1 2 3 4 N/A

11. Is there minimal use of special keys such as *control, escape,* etc.?

   1 2 3 4 N/A

12. Is hard copy output available?   1 2 3 4 N/A

13. Does the user have control over the format of the printed output?

   1 2 3 4 N/A

14. Is the user able to set the speed of screen output, including scrolling?

   1 2 3 4 N/A

15. Are there graphics capabilities available? This is very useful in spread sheets and statistical programs.   1 2 3 4 N/A

16. Is the screen layout easy to read (e.g., *not* 24 lines of single-spaced text)?

   1 2 3 4 N/A

17. Does each screen present a reasonable amount of information? Too much information on a particular screen can be confusing.   1 2 3 4 N/A

18. Is there display of upper- and lower-case characters?   1 2 3 4 N/A

19. Are new screens displayed quickly, without excessive delays?

   1 2 3 4 N/A

20. Is the text free of spelling errors?   1 2 3 4 N/A

21. Is the text free of punctuation errors?   1 2 3 4 N/A

22. Is the text grammatically correct?   1 2 3 4 N/A

23. Can the program share data with other programs from the same or different manufacturers?   1 2 3 4 N/A

24. Is this an integrated software package? That is, does it allow exchange of information with other programs, such as spread sheets using data stored in a data base or "dropping charts" from a plotting program into a word processing file?   1 2 3 4 N/A

25. Does the program employ color effectively?   1 2 3 4 N/A

26. Does the program allow easy backup of data disks? It is best if the backup routine is part of the program, since this will encourage you to back up.   1 2 3 4 N/A

27. Would the program be useful in situations other than those for which it was specifically designed?   1 2 3 4 N/A

Documentation

28. Is adequate documentation—e.g., manuals—supplied?   1 2 3 4 N/A

29. If documentation is not supplied, can it be purchased at a reasonable cost?   1 2 3 4 N/A

30. Is the documentation written clearly?   1 2 3 4 N/A

31. Does the documentation provide examples of use?   1 2 3 4 N/A

32. Does the documentation present examples of screen layouts? This is helpful in relating sections in the manual to actual applications appearing on the monitor.   1 2 3 4 N/A

33. Can the program be used without special training?   1 2 3 4 N/A

34. If a tutorial would be useful, is one provided?   1 2 3 4 N/A

35. Are the technical aspects for installing the software described? This refers to setting up the program to run on your computer, getting the printer to run correctly, etc.   1 2 3 4 N/A

36. Is there minimal need for additional materials that result in additional expense?   1 2 3 4 N/A

37. Is troubleshooting information available?   1 2 3 4 N/A

38. Are error messages explained and appropriate actions indicated?   1 2 3 4 N/A

39. Are operating instructions for various kinds of equipment described?   1 2 3 4 N/A

Sales and Support

40. Is there a support telephone number listed?   1 2 3 4 N/A

41. If a support number is listed, is it answered promptly? Some support numbers are continually busy or are never answered.   1 2 3 4 N/A

42. Is the manufacturer an established company with a good track record?   1 2 3 4 N/A

43. Are replacements for disks that won't work provided free or at a nominal charge?   1 2 3 4 N/A

44. Is there a backup copy of the program provided with the original disk, or are you allowed to make a backup copy?   1 2 3 4 N/A

45. Is there a local vendor for the manufacturer? This is most often a salesperson in a computer or software store.   1 2 3 4 N/A

46. Have you read any software reviews—in computer publications, for example—that support the claims of the manufacturer and/or vendor?   1 2 3 4 N/A

47. Contact other users. Do they express satisfaction with the product?   1 2 3 4 N/A

48. If training is necessary, can it be provided by the vendor?   1 2 3 4 N/A

49. If training is necessary, is it free?   1 2 3 4 N/A

50. Does the vendor know how to use the software as opposed to simply delivering a sales pitch?   1 2 3 4 N/A

51. If the answer to 44 is no, is there technical assistance *immediately* available from another source?   1 2 3 4 N/A

52. If you are buying from a local vendor, does the operation look respectable, that is, is it a clean, orderly showroom?   1 2 3 4 N/A

53. Are enhancements provided free or at a nominal charge (e.g., the cost of the disk)?   1 2 3 4 N/A

To score, add up the numerals circled and divide by the number of items that did not have N/A as the response.

$$Score = \frac{sum\ of\ responses}{number\ of\ items}$$

Education Software

If you are evaluating education software, ask these questions in addition to the general questions listed above.

54. Is the content appropriate to the target audience?   1 2 3 4 N/A

55. Does the instructional design—i.e., tutorial, drill and practice, etc.—complement the content?   1 2 3 4 N/A

56. Is the content factually accurate?   1 2 3 4 N/A

57. Does the program make effective use of branching? (E.g., does the program look different for a "good" student than for one encountering difficulties?)   1 2 3 4 N/A

58. Can the user review sections of the text?   1 2 3 4 N/A

59. Does the program allow string input (words or phrases) as opposed to simply letters or numbers?   1 2 3 4 N/A

Software Evaluation Checklist, continued

60. Does the software take full advantage of the educational capabilities of the computer versus simple "page turning"?   1 2 3 4 N/A

61. Does use of the computer enhance teaching of the topic?   1 2 3 4 N/A

62. Are the instructional strategies, goals, and objectives clearly explained?   1 2 3 4 N/A

63. Is the lesson content congruent with goals and objectives?   1 2 3 4 N/A

64. Is the lesson structure directed at mastery learning?   1 2 3 4 N/A

65. Are instructional prerequisites described?   1 2 3 4 N/A

66. If appropriate, are instructional prerequisites tested?   1 2 3 4 N/A

67. Is the length of the lesson appropriate to the audience's attention span?   1 2 3 4 N/A

68. Is there a pretest?   1 2 3 4 N/A

69. Does the user control presentation of content, e.g., by being directed to "press a key to continue"?   1 2 3 4 N/A

70. Are relevant examples provided?   1 2 3 4 N/A

71. Are examples randomly selected?   1 2 3 4 N/A

72. Are questions and/or problems randomly generated?   1 2 3 4 N/A

73. Is feedback immediate?   1 2 3 4 N/A

74. Is feedback appropriate to the response?   1 2 3 4 N/A

75. Is feedback noncondescending?   1 2 3 4 N/A

76. Is feedback randomized?   1 2 3 4 N/A

77. Are diagnostics available to identify student problems? That is, does the program keep record of student responses in order to pinpoint problems as the student goes through the lesson?   1 2 3 4 N/A

78. Is there a posttest?   1 2 3 4 N/A

79. Do the tests assess the goals and objectives of the lesson?   1 2 3 4 N/A

80. If tests can be generated, is the total number of items under your control (versus the program dictating the maximum number of items)?   1 2 3 4 N/A

81. Is management of student records available?   1 2 3 4 N/A

82. If there is a management system, is it simple to use?   1 2 3 4 N/A

83. Is student privacy protected?   1 2 3 4 N/A

Software Evaluation Checklist, continued

84. Can enough student records be stored to be of practical use?　　　　　　　　1 2 3 4 N/A

85. If graphics are used, do they enhance learning?　　　1 2 3 4 N/A

86. If video (as in videocassette or videodisk) is used, does it enhance learning?　　　　1 2 3 4 N/A

87. If audio is used, does it enhance learning?　　　1 2 3 4 N/A

88. If the software package contains numerous lessons, is there a hierarchical structure? A hierarchical structure would allow students to progress (skip lessons based on meeting pretest criteria) or regress (review previous material that has not been learned) at their own pace.　　1 2 3 4 N/A

89. Is there any suggestion of how to integrate the software into the overall curriculum?　　　1 2 3 4 N/A

90. Can the instructor modify the program for specific lessons or teaching situations?　　　1 2 3 4 N/A

91. Can the instructor modify the program for new equipment, students, etc.?　　　1 2 3 4 N/A

92. Are additional instructional activities suggested?　　　1 2 3 4 N/A

To score this section, add up the numerals circled and divide by the number of items which did not have N/A as the response.

$$Score = \frac{sum\ of\ responses}{number\ of\ items}$$

Total score = general section + education score.

The total score should allow you to compare a number of packages.

Assuring Quality
in Nursing
Education

STRATEGIES FOR RECRUITING GRADUATE FACULTY IN NURSING SERVICE ADMINISTRATION

JOAN O'LEARY, RN, EdD
Associate Professor, College of Nursing
Graduate Program, Villanova University
Villanova, Pennsylvania

There is a great need for prepared nursing service administrators. These truly may be the best of best times for the profession of nursing, or the worst of worst times. The advent of diagnosis-related groups (DRGs) has created an increased need for prepared nurses to assume the top executive position within the health care system. Our ability to survive in the nursing profession rests on our ability to organize human beings in such a way as to generate opportunity and results, rather than impasse, stagnation, and wasteful friction. The old approaches in nursing management can lead to our demise. The role of those in nursing management must become enriched through education and through authority and responsibility made rational.

Nursing administration theory encompasses both nursing and management. To broaden and prepare the nursing administrators of tomorrow, curricula must include substantive knowledge inside and outside the discipline of nursing. The art of managing people is multidimensional and, to date, is not included in many textbooks. Nursing management can encompass everything from data acquisition to computerization of systems to performance evaluation to complex organizational dynamics to implementing nursing theory.

The only way to gain control of the health care system is to fill its ranks with prepared, competent nursing administrators. Individuals must stand up and be counted, and they must control and manage the human resources within their institutions. This is the only way needs for high quality health care will be met.

There are many power groups within the health arena, all vying for control. Hospital administrators, boards of trustees, medical staffs, financial and legal officers frequently would like to control the nursing system, and some now do. If we do not prepare individuals who will assume the responsibility for nursing administration, someone else will. The quality of care in the health arena depends on the knowledge that a nursing administrator brings to an institution. These individuals must determine the processes and strategies needed to achieve standards within an organization.

ROLE OF NURSING ADMINISTRATORS

The role of those in nursing administration must be defined and their authority and responsibility made rational. The control and authority that traditionally has resided with boards of directors and chief operating officers should rest in the department of nursing. If nursing administrators are prepared, positive contributions and positive direction will result.

Those in nursing administration should know full well that much of their success depends on their relationships with medical staffs and hospital administration. To achieve these relationships requires one to be astute politically, understand the principles of power, and know management.

Some nursing administrators, because of their lack of knowledge or their lack of power, are willing to give up their overall responsibility for nursing. The reaction of one director of nursing when her department was placed under the engineering department was, "That's okay— at least I have a job." In nursing, we have given up so much. Physical therapists now do range of motion, respiratory therapists now comfortably handle respiratory care, social workers do discharge planning. Do we now comfortably relinquish our authority to an engineering department? This authority and responsibility must not be relinquished!

It is our responsibility to prepare knowledgeable, competent leaders— individuals who are not only oriented toward nursing theory, but are prepared in finance as well as in management. These individuals not only need to be prepared in the theoretical arena, they also must know the practical, down-to-earth strategies and the "how-to" in order to change and progress in a positive fashion.

How can a nursing administrator truly analyze and synthesize organizational dynamics without being prepared by those who have been there? Nursing administrators desperately need strong role models. Many have learned by trial and error, and for many it has been learning the hard way. Education of these individuals must rest in the graduate educational arena. Their teachers must have not only the needed educational preparation but also experience through which they can relate the scanty theory to practice. Teaching administration without practitioners in administration can be compared to reading a manual to learn how to change a tire. You can read and memorize; but it isn't until the fateful day when the tire blows that you realize that you may know "how-to," but you should also have *practiced* "how-to."

Those in nursing administration should be comfortable with involvement in policy development and the decision-making processes that directly affect nursing practice within a system. These individuals must have didactic content as well as an in-depth knowledge of the political processes at the federal, state, and local level. Administrators should not only be extremely aware of the current national trends within the profession, but they also must assume a key role in influencing the legislative and political processes that directly affect the profession and consumers of health care.

If we are to survive, it is imperative that executives be prepared to function actively and from a position of legitimate authority and power.[1] How does one attain that position? It is evident from the Magnet Hospital Study that individuals need to be prepared in administration, in professional practice, and in the area of professional development.[2] These educational requirements exist not only at the executive level, but for all of those within the management arena in the health care system. Leaders do not function alone, but succeed only with a cadre of competent, prepared subordinates.

How can students preparing for nursing administration roles within health care agencies know and recognize the uniqueness of this knowledge base without having before them strong, knowledgeable, competent leaders as teachers and role models? Those in education must assume the responsibility for preparing the future leaders in nursing administration. Schools of nursing must seek faculty who are prepared educationally and administratively. It is these experienced administrators who will provide the leadership and direction for this valuable and needed discipline.

There is an intense need to further study and define what is needed for success in the field of nursing administration. The role is evolving, and at the same time schools of nursing are beginning to establish graduate programs to prepare those in nursing management. Curricula must be identified and courses established that will meet the demands of the position. Deans and faculty within schools of nursing should consider meeting these challenges by adopting a blueprint or a marketing strategy to recruit viable faculty to ensure that upon graduation individuals will be prepared for their role in nursing administration.

---

[1] National Commission on Nursing, *Initial Report and Preliminary Recommendations* (Chicago, Il.: Hospital Research and Educational Trust, September 1981).

[2] Task Force on Nursing Practice in Hospitals, *Magnet Hospitals: Attraction and Retention of Professional Nurses* (Kansas City, Mo.: American Academy of Nursing, 1983).

STRATEGIES FOR RECRUITING FACULTY

How can one hire prepared faculty to meet the challenge of preparing students for nursing administration? What can deans and faculty do to recruit available experienced faculty members to develop and teach in these programs? The following are some strategies that can be utilized to recruit experienced faculty.

Sell Yourself and Your Program. Deans and faculty who are interested in attracting qualified faculty members should make the time to meet individuals in leadership roles throughout the country. Many professional organizations support the nursing service administrator.

The National Forum for Administrators of Nursing of the National League for Nursing is an executive group for administrators. Membership provides an active forum for administrators, with annual meetings and many educational programs. For example, this group recently conducted a program on marketing skills. Any dean or faculty member could have attended, gained from the program, and at the same time searched for the new qualified faculty.

To become a full member of the American Society for Administrators of Nursing of the American Hospital Association, one must be the chief or associate chief in nursing. Those responsible for a graduate program in nursing administration are eligible for associate membership. The society has yearly conventions, usually attended by five to seven thousand nursing administrators, and their programs are also excellent. The contacts and networks formed at these conventions can facilitate the recruitment of qualified faculty.

Negotiate Good Salaries. Many in graduate education are concerned with the dichotomy that exists between salaries in the hospitals and those in the universities. Universities have to recognize that qualified administrators who may be earning high salaries may be difficult to recruit. An imaginative dean can recruit such administrators by offering the best salaries that they can negotiate and, at the same time, offering flexibility in scheduling class and committee time. Offer administrators "free days" so that their time can be utilized for research, consultation, and publication. Successful administrators can actually increase their salaries, if they have the imagination and drive to do so.

Encourage Joint Practice. Those in administration can be recruited by encouraging faculty to practice while teaching. All schools of nursing have developed strong relationships in the hospital and home care arenas that are vital for undergraduate programs. Many of these institutions might be interested in hiring on a part-time basis someone teaching in administration. Salaries could be negotiated between the two agencies, and joint or collaborative relationships could be beneficial for both groups.

Sell Research. The field of nursing administration is dramatically lacking in research data. Those who work in this field must identify problems and, through proper analysis, more clearly delineate the role and scope of practice in nursing administration. Research in this field should focus on critically analyzing the social, ethical, and political forces important to the discipline of administration. Further defining and analyzing the role of those in administration could be a rewarding and worthwhile experience.

Offer the Ability to Publish. A full-time associate professorship requires taking or making time to publish and to contribute to the profession through presentations. Those who are actively teaching really can accomplish their teaching responsibilities in 30 hours. They may still have 50 hours left over in which to do all the things that they have wanted to do, yet never had the time for when working 80 hours a week. Publishing as a faculty member can generate a sense of satisfaction and accomplishment without the feeling of having to neglect your job to do so.

Encourage Consultation. Successful administrators can expand their scope of practice through consultation to health care agencies. A formalized administrative contract can be a viable mechanism for improving the entire health care delivery system.

Successful administrators are often limited in expanding their impact to the entire health arena because they are committed to their own institution. The innovations they carry out usually stay within one institution. A teacher can increase his or her visibility through student contacts. If consultation results, the teacher then has the opportunity to put into practice what she preaches at a variety of institutions and to contribute in a wider fashion than if she had stayed at the hospital.

The newest criteria for accreditation of graduate programs by the NLN encourages faculty practice. Villanova University, for one, encourages such adventures. The dean encourages faculty to maintain their expertise and gives them the freedom to be creative and innovative. In return, faculty members can provide written descriptions of their activities.

Offer Tenure. Experts in administration who are educationally prepared may arrive at the university with diverse backgrounds. Faculty members who participate on tenure committees might establish such rigorous tenure requirements that these administrators are unable to meet them. Their research may not be considered intense enough, their publications not scholarly. Deans of schools of nursing may have to use political clout to facilitate the tenure process for administrators.

Sell Job Security. Tenure implies job security. Of course, if the number of graduate students decline and the pool dries up, greener pastures have to be sought, but as long as students have educational needs and those needs are met, job security exists. How many administrators can really attest to having that kind of security?

Those in nursing administration often don't know from one day to the next whether they will have a job. They are at the mercy of hospital administrators and medical staffs. Of course, at the university one is responsible to the dean, but as a faculty member, I have the academic freedom to meet the course objectives in the manner that I feel is appropriate. The administrative relationship that exists between faculty and university administration is significantly different than that which exists within the hierarchy of the hospital. True, if one does not uphold the philosophy of the university, one may be fired, but the chances of that happening rest with the individual and not with others.

Sell Flexible, Realistic Hours. I alluded earlier to the intense workload of those in nursing administration. Those who are effective in that world have learned to manage their time efficiently just to survive. Many of those in nursing have personal responsibilities over and above the job. To survive the pressures, those in management may neglect those valuable personal responsibilities, not intentionally, but because they do not have the time to take care of everyone.

A teaching schedule, however, is flexible. It allows you to meet with a sixth-grade teacher for counseling of a youngster. The teaching schedule does not require punching a time clock. A faculty member does not have to justify his or her time or demonstrate that she or he has worked eight straight hours. The position requires teaching certain courses, participating in committees, advising students, practicing, publishing, and conducting research. When all is said and done, you manage your own time. When you are not required to be at school, no one ever asks where you have been. The freedom allowed to faculty exists throughout the university. The faculty member is treated as a mature individual who is expected to meet the objectives of the overall program.

Sell Collegial Relationships. The university abounds with creative, innovative, dynamic thinkers. Those who have migrated to that environment are usually intelligent, interested people. Informal debates with other faculty members over an idea or a concept are common. Some of the discussions have encouraged me to view the sociological perspective, the psychological perspective, or the nursing perspective. In most health care institutions, in contrast, the top person might have a master's degree, and some staff members might be attending school. Often, because of lack of colleagues to provide stimulating feedback or lack of time, that environment is not conducive to the development of concepts vital to the managment processes. Successful enterprises are lead by those who have the time to be imaginative and creative. A solid sounding board is necessary for innovations in health care.

Encourage Full-Time Administrators to Teach Part Time. Many administrators are gratified to have the opportunity to teach and work with students. These administrators have the opportunity to bring the real world into the classroom. The university can offer them a salary as well as an opportunity to recharge their own thinking processes.

Tell the World That You are Looking for That Outstanding Faculty Member. There are many publications—from the *New York Times* to the *Journal of Nursing Service Administration*—that can put your needs before the public. If you offer freedom, creativeness, and challenges, you might be positively surprised when quality curricula vitae arrive in front of you.

Let your faculty know that you are in need of additional teachers. If your faculty know that the search committee is looking for a qualified administrator, they can begin expanding their networks in order to identify potential candidates.

Sell Satisfaction and an Expanding Network. No one really ever praises the nursing administrator. He or she is simply expected to be the be-all and end-all of everything. Providing the teacher meets the course objectives, students often offer positive feedback to a faculty member. Having a student say; "I really do not understand," or "I tried that strategy and it worked" sometimes is worth all the money in the world. Much satisfaction comes from the relationships that are built within the classroom. In the years to come, those students who have passed through my classroom will maintain that closeness and that comradeship. I also have the satisfaction of knowing that I am part of a force that will contribute to molding our profession. Along with other faculty members I have helped to salvage a part of the profession. The future leaders in nursing that we have prepared are competent to tackle the health care industry, and they will shape nursing in the decades ahead.

CREDENTIALING: THE THREAD BETWEEN LICENSURE, ACCREDITATION, AND CERTIFICATION

ROBERT V. PIEMONTE, EdD, RN
Director of the Division of House, Board,
and Cabinet Affairs
American Nurses' Association
Kansas City, Missouri

Credentialing refers to the process of accreditation, licensure, and certification, and discussion of the subject should encompass all three elements. Accreditation, a crucial component of the entire process, is often disregarded as we attempt to deal with regulation of advanced practice through the credentialing mechanism of certification.

It is important to understand that the accreditation of our education programs in nursing is interrelated with the mechanisms of licensure and certification. All three mechanisms assist in assuring the quality of nursing care to the publics we serve. Through credentialing mechanisms, the profession maintains standards of education and service and stimulates continued self-improvement of nursing practitioners.

The fundamental components of credentialing are quality, identity, protection, and control. Professionals recognize accreditation, certification, licensure, and academic degrees as mechanisms designed to assure quality, thereby protecting the public. Although credentialing serves to confer occupational identity, it essentially operates to protect the public from substandard practices.

LICENSURE

It is appropriate to begin the discussion of credentialing with licensure since it is the oldest of all credentialing mechanisms used in this country to regulate a profession. The report of the American Nurses' Association

Committee on the Study of Credentialing in Nursing recommended a
definition of licensure that encompasses elements about which, I believe,
all can agree:

> Licensure is a process by which an agency of state government
> grants permission to individuals accountable for the practice of a
> profession to engage in the practice of that profession and prohibits
> all others from legally doing so. It permits use of a particular title.
> Its purpose is to protect the public by ensuring a minimum level
> of professional competence. Established standards and methods of
> evaluation are used to determine eligibility for initial licensure and
> for periodic renewal. Effective means are employed for taking ac-
> tion against licensees for acts of professional misconduct, in-
> competence, and/or negligence.[1]

History of Legal Regulation

It may be surprising to learn that Florence Nightingale was an oppo-
nent of examination and registration for the practice of nursing. In the
late nineteenth century, she opposed the British Nurses Association in its
efforts to obtain a royal charter that would permit it to test and register
nurses. Nightingale believed that a focus on the competence of nurses rather
than on character would destroy her work to upgrade the profession's social
and moral standards. Fortunately, Nightingale's opposition did not deter
the efforts of Ethel Gordon Bedford Fenwick, founder of the British Nurses
Association. Her campaign for registration of nurses stimulated early leaders
of nursing in the United States to seek registration and uniform standards
of nursing education. The movement was spearheaded by the Associated
Alumnae of Trained Nurses of the United States and Canada, founded
in 1897. This organization was later renamed the American Nurses'
Association.

The campaign for registration gained momentum from 1898 to 1901
with the formation of state nurses' associations. The *American Journal of
Nursing* strove to rally support for registration and published samples of
draft legislation. In 1903, North Carolina became the first state to enact
a registration law. In the same year, New Jersey, New York, and Virginia
followed suit.

Although the laws varied in language and specifications, most included
three basic provisions. First, untrained nurses were denied use of the title
"registered nurse." Second, the laws established a mechanism for examining
training school graduates. Third, they established a "grandfathering"
process—a period of time during which qualified trained nurses were eligible
to register without examination.

Over the next 20 years, each of the 48 states, plus Hawaii and the
District of Columbia, enacted legislation affecting nurse training. There

[1] *The Study of Credentialing in Nursing: A New Approach* (Kansas City, Mo.: American Nurses' Association, 1979).

were problems, however. The legislation was diverse and, therefore, inconsistent. Ambiguity in the language of the laws and indifference from some training schools and nurses made it difficult for early boards of nursing to administer the acts. Some qualified nurses failed to apply for registration. Because states lacked experience in constructing examinations, questions were often ambiguous and examination results were questionable. The most serious problem was the failure of the legislation to define nursing practice and to limit it to those qualified.

In 1915, ANA began actively assisting state associations in the campaign for licensure. The association drafted a model law to serve as a reference to states pursuing registration laws. ANA worked with the National League of Nursing Education to examine licensure in 41 jurisdictions and issued a statement endorsing compulsory licensure for "all those who nurse for hire."

To protect both the public and the profession from unqualified practitioners, it was essential to define the scope of nursing practice. New York was successful in adopting a compulsory law with a definition of nursing practice in 1938. Similar efforts in other areas received both opposition and support. Resistance came from hospital administrators. The movement was delayed by the acute shortage of nurses during World War II—a shortage that also brought about full recognition of practical nurses. Stratification of nursing roles gave support to the arguments of registered nurses in support of mandatory licensure.

Meanwhile, nurses were increasing their roles in diagnostic and therapeutic decision making. The emergence of advanced clinical specialties pointed up the need for further revision of nursing practice acts. Nurses were engaging in actions that were outside the legally defined scope of their practice. Idaho was the first state to accommodate the change in nursing practice by amending its act in 1971 to include language authorizing nursing diagnosis and treatment.

ANA Policy on Licensure

The ANA publication, *Nursing: A Social Policy Statement*, was developed to define the social context of professional nursing practice.[2] The statement describes a contract between nursing and society, under which society grants status, authority, and control over practice to nursing. In return, it is the nurse's duty to practice in a manner that maintains the public trust. Licensure laws are a concrete example of this contract. These laws are commonly referred to as nursing practice acts. Although no two are alike, they share a common purpose: to protect the public. Through licensure, the public is guaranteed minimum standards for entry into the profession and guaranteed a way to identify the unqualified.

---

[2] *Nursing: A Social Policy Statement* (Kansas City, Mo.: American Nurses' Association, 1980).

The American Nurses' Association has always been concerned about and involved in issues of licensure. ANA has endorsed the following six basic principles relating to the legal regulation of nursing practice:

1. ANA believes the primary purpose of a licensing law is to protect the public health and welfare by establishing legal qualifications for nursing practice. Such qualifications are recognized as minimum standards necessary to provide safe and effective nursing practice.

2. ANA believes all persons practicing or offering to practice nursing or practical nursing should be licensed. The public can be protected only if all who practice nursing are licensed. The public should not be expected to differentiate between incompetent and competent practitioners.

3. ANA believes that since nursing is one occupational field, there should be one nursing practice act that licenses both registered nurses and licensed practical nurses. The public and members of the profession may become confused if more than one law regulates the practice of nursing and the practice of practical nursing.

4. The enactment of one nursing practice act requires only one licensing board for nursing in a state. The board of nursing should be composed of nurses whose practice is regulated by the licensure law and by a representative or representatives of the public.

5. Candidates for licensure should complete an educational program approved by the board and pass the licensing examination before a license to practice is granted.

6. The nursing practice act should provide for the legal regulation of nursing without reference to a specialized area of practice. ANA believes it is the function of the professional association to establish the scope and desirable qualifications required for each area of practice and to certify individuals as competent to engage in specialized practice. It is also the function of the professional association to upgrade practice above the minimum standards set by laws. The law should not provide for identifying clinical specialists in nursing or require certification or other recognition for practice beyond the minimum qualifications for the legal regulation of nursing.

Status of Nursing Practice Acts

Nursing practice acts vary in their conformity to these principles. They also vary widely in their approaches to defining the legal scope of nursing practice.

Each jurisdiction in the United States, with the exception of the District of Columbia, provides a definition of nursing practice within its practice act. The definition identifies the components of nursing practice, which should suffice as the legal scope of nursing practice. Unfortunately for nursing, legislators have added other provisions in the definitions of nursing practice or elsewhere in the law that significantly affect the legal scope of nursing practice.

Additional provisions in nursing practice acts fall into three categories: (1) specific sections within the law addressing specialized nursing practice; (2) blanket prohibitions against medical diagnosis and treatment; and (3) clauses that permit performance of additional acts by specially trained nurses as authorized by board of nursing rules. The addition of these clauses has resulted in the development of specific rules regulating the scope of advanced or specialized nursing practice.

The ANA has developed a model definition of nursing practice, which was first issued by the Congress for Nursing Practice.[3] The definition describes the knowledge base required for the practice of nursing and the traditional five steps of the nursing process. It also describes the components of nursing practice in broad language that would not be restrictive to nursing's evolving scope of practice. The ANA model definition emphasizes that each of us is accountable for the quality of care we give.

Although the terms *licensure* and *registration* are often used synonymously, their meanings are quite different. The ANA Committee for the Study of Credentialing in Nursing defined registration as

> a process by which qualified individuals are listed on an official roster maintained by a governmental or non-governmental agency. It enables such persons to use a particular title and attests to employing agencies and individuals that minimum qualifications have been met and maintained.[4]

ACCREDITATION

National voluntary accreditation is recognized as a means to ensure the provision of high-quality education in the United States. In this country, responsibility for education is presumed to be a state's right. Therefore, although voluntary accrediting agencies have no legal power, their actions are recognized as reliable indicators of an institution's merits. A perfect case in point is the influence that accreditation by the National League for Nursing—or the lack thereof—has on graduates seeking admission to graduate programs in nursing.

Accreditation agencies such as the National League for Nursing have attained quasi-governmental power. This power has been accorded by federal and state governments because these organizations have been

---

[3] *The Nursing Practice Act: Suggested State Legislation* (Kansas City, Mo.: American Nurses' Association, 1980).

[4] *The Study of Credentialing in Nursing.*

determined to be reliable agents in identifying institutions having meritorious programs of study. Voluntary accreditation has been used by government agencies to satisfy legal requirements rather than establish duplicative mechanisms. Consequently, all of us in education have a vested interest in the process.

The definition of accreditation suggested by the ANA Committee on the Study of Credentialing in Nursing encompasses those elements necessary to an effective accreditation process. The committee described accreditation as

> the process by which a voluntary, non-governmental agency or organization appraises and grants accredited status to institutions and/or programs or services which meet predetermined structure, process, and outcome criteria. Its purposes are to evaluate the performance of a service or educational program and to provide to various publics information upon which to base decisions about the utilization of the institutions, programs, services, and/or graduates. Periodic assessment is an integral part of the accreditation process in order to ensure continual acceptable performance. Accreditation is conducted by agencies which have been recognized or approved by an organized peer group of agencies as having integrity and consistency in their practices.[5]

It is important to remember that there are two types of educational accreditation: institutional and programmatic. Nursing accreditation performed by the National League for Nursing is program accreditation, also referred to as professional accreditation. Accreditation has been the most valuable credentialing mechanism in upgrading the quality of nursing education. This development has had a positive effect on the quality of nursing care delivered.

The interrelatedness of accreditation with the mechanisms of licensure and certification was noted earlier. Licensure is intended to ensure safe nursing care, and accreditation is intended to raise the quality of care through education. Whereas licensure promotes minimum safe practice, accreditation seeks to promote excellence. Accreditation assures a quality beyond that required of the institution for approval by the state. Accreditation should not be confused with approval, which is a process used to designate a nursing school's competence to prepare practitioners.

Although all the credentialing mechanisms are fraught with problems, the most effective quality-assurance mechanism available for schools of nursing is self-regulation through voluntary accreditation.

CERTIFICATION

The last credentialing mechanism to be discussed is certification, which

---

[5] *Ibid.*

attests to an individual's attainment of predetermined skills and knowledge in a specific field of study. Referring once again to ANA's study of credentialing in nursing, certification is defined as

> a process by which a non-governmental agency or association cer- tifies that an individual licensed to practice a profession has met certain predetermined standards specified by that profession for speciality practice. Its purpose is to assure various publics that an individual has mastered a body of knowledge and acquired skills in a particular specialty.[6]

The term has meaning when used in connection with a particular specialty—for example, nurse midwife or nurse anesthetist. Prestige is associated with certification because of the special knowledge and skill required. Since the the knowledge and skill required exceeds what is needed to become licensed, the number of people certified in a specialty are a minority in a profession. The interrelatedness of all three creden- tialing mechanisms is again evidenced in examining the main objective of certification: to ensure that the public receives quality nursing care. However, certification serves several other objectives. It encourages specialization and advanced practice and in some instances provides a vehicle for the reimbursement of nurses. Although certification in nursing is relatively new when compared to licensure, it is providing practitioners with the opportunity to upgrade their practice with a minimum of government interference.

The Study of Credentialing in Nursing describes the differences between the priorities of certification and those of licensure and accreditation as follows:

> Licensure, while attesting to an individual's capability to meet a set of legal requirements, concentrates on the public's right to pro- tection. Accreditation is designed exclusively for institutions and programs and attests to their base level of quality. Certification, as a professional voluntary credentialing mechanism, attests to the profession's recognition of an individual's competence for advanced or specialized practice, applied toward the ultimate benefit of the public and institutions. From this perspective, certification may be seen as establishing a balance within the triangle of interplaying interests involved in credentialing, that is, the interests of the public, those of the institutions, and now, those of the individual professional.[7]

The future of all credentialing mechanisms depends on the profes-

---

[6] *Ibid.*

[7] *Ibid.*

sion's ability to develop a unified system for these activities. Independence from government control hinges on our readiness to regulate our practice.

PROBLEMS IN SELF-REGULATION

Although the information presented here may be interesting and even helpful from a historical perspective, questions must be raised about nursing's progress in the credentialing arena. As noted earlier, all the credentialing mechanisms have problems. To examine ways in which the profession might progress, current problems have to be addressed or, at the very least, examined.

One of the basic hallmarks of any profession is self-regulation. Without that authority, the collective becomes a trade group whose standards, codes, beliefs, and the like are determined by others. The self-regulatory responsibility of the profession is that it requires minimum external regulation and exercises minimum self-regulation in the public interest. Boards of nursing within the states provide this public interest protection by promulgating rules and regulations that govern the broad role of the nurse. It is the responsibility of the profession—nurses in an organized collective—to define, implement, evaluate, and refine the major regulations of practice. The nursing profession derives its authority for its practice from society; we exist because society has determined that there is a demonstrable need for our service. This pact that nursing has with society also is a contract from society to nursing.

Our part of the social contract is the activities that nursing must engage in as a collective in carrying out the profession's responsibility to society. They include:

1. Establishing a code of ethics.
2. Establishing standards of practice.
3. Fostering the development of nursing theory to explain observations and guide nursing actions.
4. Establishing educational requirements for entry into professional practice.
5. Developing certification processes for the profession.
6. Other developmental work directed toward making more specific nursing's accountability to society.

One of the consequences of these and other self-regulatory activities of nursing has been enactment of nursing practice acts and related licensure legislation and regulations that make specific the legal authority to practice. This legal authority to practice stems from the social contract between society and the profession; the social contract does not derive from legislation.

The certification and accreditation mechanisms of credentialing are the property of the profession of nursing. Currently these responsibilities are carried out by a variety of organizations, including the American Nurses' Association, the National League for Nursing, and some specialty nursing organizations.

Certification

Certification has been defined as an instrument whereby a professional organization can attest that an individual has attained proficiency in an area of that profession's practice. That sounds like a simple enough description. However, if one looks more closely at how certification in the profession has been used, a far more complex picture emerges. It appears that certification can be for entry into practice or for validation of competence; it can be used for recognition of excellence or for regulation; it can be mandatory, academic, or professional. Assuming a common generic definition and use of certification is virtually impossible at this time, in part because we keep changing our definitions. Certification represents a relatively new credentialing mechanism for nursing. For many allied health occupations, certification has served as an entry credential for practice. In medicine, specialty certification initially was defined as a means for recognizing excellence. Today, it is a widely accepted and utilized measure for minimum professional competence in a specialty.

In the nursing profession, certification has generally served as a means of attesting to one's proficiency beyond initial licensure. In a few instances, such as the case of nurse midwives and nurse anesthetists, certification in nursing came to be recognized more as an entry credential for specialty practice. Certification affords the profession a means to attest to the qualifications of the members of the profession. It has been defined as one measure of the continued competency of individuals and as a means of documenting, to some extent, continued professional development. It is hoped that certification will serve as a process to encourage the individual's accountability for growth in his or her own practice. In addition, the certification process enables a profession to define and articulate for its members the new knowledge required for practice.

The uncertainties about certification trouble not only members of our profession, but also the public we serve. We must continue to examine the issues and answer the questions if we and the public are to reap the full benefits that this credentialing mechanism can offer.

Licensure: Nursing Practice Acts

If certification is besieged with uncertainties, licensure presents a host of problems in relation to advanced nursing practice and the profession's ability to regulate its own practice. Last year, Clare LaBar, of the ANA staff, reviewed 51 nursing practice acts to compare laws against the association's principles and model definition of nursing practice.[8] The results of the comparision indicated that every state, with the exception of Ohio, has a statutory definition of nursing that includes a general description or listing of what nursing practice is. The listing of acts or functions can have limiting interpretations and can restrict nursing practice. ANA recommends that definitions of nursing contain open-ended, flexible language that will permit the evolution of nursing practice as our profession develops.

Two major problems are apparent from the analysis of the definitions of nursing practice in nursing practice acts. The first is that the functional components of nursing are often presented as exclusive, leaving no consideration of other functions. The second problem is that the definitions of functional components often are not in broad enough terms to allow for movement and growth. These restrictions are detrimental to nursing, particularly at this time of rapidly evolving roles. In the mid-fifties, ANA advised state nurses' associations to insert a disclaimer at the end of statutory definitions of nursing practice. The disclaimer indicated that the foregoing definition should "not be deemed to include acts of diagnosis or prescription of therapeutic or corrective measures." Many states added this disclaimer until, in 1965, ANA advised that it be removed. Today, however, the disclaimer can still be found in the definitions of eight states. The only change in the disclaimer has been the insertion of the word "medical" before "diagnosis and prescription."

The use of disclaimers to definitions of nursing practice has the potential to restrict the practice of nursing. In contrast, some state definitions include language that may permit development of specialized roles and practices. Language in the Colorado act refers to "prevention, diagnosis, and treatment of human disease, ailment, pain." The Connecticut act refers to "collaborating in the implementation of the total health care regimen."

A number of state nursing practice acts include additional acts clauses. Such clauses describe the performance of additional acts by specially trained nurses. ANA policy specifically prohibits such clauses because it believes that the professional association should establish the scope and qualifications of each specialized area of practice. The development of additional acts clauses can be traced to the late 1960s and early 1970s, when nursing roles began to evolve, particularly in primary health care and nurse midwifery. Nurses practicing in new roles felt uncertain of their legal position and experienced pressure from the medical community. They, in turn, put pressure on professional associations to change

---

[8] Clare LaBar, "Legal Regulation of Nursing Practice." Paper presented at the Conference on Certification and Assessment of Professional Competence: Toward an Improved Credentialing System in Nursing, San Antonio, Texas, March 1-2, 1984.

existing laws to allow for the performance of additional acts. Today, 24 state nursing practice acts have additional acts clauses. Their existence has caused three troublesome situations for nursing.

The first problem is that additional acts clauses set the stage for legal recognition of advanced levels of practice through the statute or the rules. Again, ANA's policy is that recognition of specialty practice and upgrading of practice above minimum legal standards are functions of the professional association.

The second problem is that additional acts clauses involve another profession in defining nursing's scope of practice. Sixteen of the 24 additional acts clauses require organized medicine's involvement in determining the legal scope of nursing practice. The involvement of another profession means that nursing has relinquished some of its control of nursing practice.

The third problem of additional acts clauses is the existence of accompanying rules to identify specific acts or practices that may be performed. The rules may be so specific as to restrict the expansion and evolution of specialty practice. They may also have the effect of prohibiting specific practices by all nurses who are not credentialed according to the law.

Additional acts clauses followed by the development of rules for specific advanced practice areas have resulted in a majority of jurisdictions' regulating specific areas of advanced practice. The rules generally prescribe a method of credentialing the advanced practitioner. In addition, boards of nursing cite specific requirements for engaging in advanced practice. These requirements vary from state to state and often from practitioner to practitioner within states. Such requirements limit the interstate mobility of nurses while adding to the administrative load of the boards of nursing.

Sometimes, administrative rules specify the scope of practice for advanced practitioners. Many scope-of-practice statements list activities that may be performed independently and those to be performed under the direction and supervision of a physician. The description of a scope of practice for advanced nursing practice is inappropriate and contrary to ANA policy. Moreover, it may have the effect of limiting the evolution of specialty practice as well as placing the practitioner in a dependent role. Development of rules for specialized practice is not as serious a problem as the inclusion of specific provisions for specialty practice in nursing practice acts. Some nursing practice acts refer to specialty practice and its content in specific sections of the law. These provisions generally specify requirements for practice acts that the nurse is permitted to perform and requirements for medical supervision or protocols.

ANA specifically prohibits statutorily defining advanced practice. Moreover, the association cautions against listing specific acts or practices in the legal definition of nursing. Those states in violation of these principles may find that their laws fail to accommodate changes in nursing practice.

Despite the prevalence of restrictive language in nursing practice acts, there is cause for optimism about the future of legal regulation of nursing practice. In recent years, many states have begun evaluating their statutory definitions of nursing practice. Recent amendments to nursing laws better reflect nursing's focus on human responses to health problems. Several nursing practice acts state that nurses diagnose and treat human responses to health problems. A few nurses' associations, such as Arizona, Florida, and Massachusetts, are looking at ways to remove from the law language regulating advanced practitioners. They believe, as ANA does, that such language may restrict the practice of nurses.

In the future, we anticipate less involvement of the medical profession in board of nursing rules for advanced practice and in advisory committees for advanced practice. More recent rules for advanced practice and requirements for advisory committees do not include the specific involvement of medicine. However, medicine continues to challenge rule development by boards of nursing, the practice of individual nurses, third-party reimbursement of nursing services, hospital privileges, and prescription-writing authority.

A recent challenge against nursing practice in Missouri yielded an important decision in support of broadly worded definitions of nursing practice. The Missouri nurse practice act was revised in 1975 to reflect the expanded role of nursing practice. In 1981, the Missouri State Board of Registration for the Healing Arts charged two nurse practitioners in a rural family planning clinic with the unauthorized practice of medicine. A St. Louis County circuit court upheld the board's action. The controversial services provided by the nurse practitioners included breast and pelvic examinations; laboratory testing of pap smears, gonorrhea cultures, and blood serology; provision of birth control devices and information; the administration of designated medication; and counseling and education services.

When the nurse practitioners appealed the decision of the circuit court, the Missouri Supreme Court reversed the lower court's decision. The State Supreme Court noted that the Missiouri nurse practice act reflected a legislative intent to "expand the scope of nursing practice." It found significant the "legislature's formulation of an open-ended definition of professional nursing." The court also concluded that the "broadening of the field of practice of the nursing profession authorized by the legislature and here recognized by the Court carries with it the profession's responsibility for continuing education standards and the individual nurse's responsibility to conduct himself or herself in a professional manner."

We can expect additional challenges to advanced nursing practice. Organized nursing has a responsibility to break medicine's informational and ideological monopoly of the health care marketplace. In addition, we have a responsibility to educate consumers about the appropriate roles and functions of nurses. Both licensure and certification are tools to assist us in achieving our goal.

Accreditation

Finally, accreditation is not without its problems. A critical issue facing accrediting agencies is innovation in educational programs. The differences among programs produces new challenges for accrediting agencies. The ANA credentialing study identified the following issues in the accreditation of nursing programs:

1. Proliferation of agencies involved in accreditation of nursing education programs.
2. Diverse systems of nursing education.
3. Spiraling costs of education.
4. Conflicts between programmatic and institutional accrediting agencies.
5. Difficulties encountered by accrediting agencies in seeking both governmental and nongovernmental approval or recognition as a credentialing agency.
6. Increasing incorporation of sociopolitical concerns pertaining to human rights, public accountability, consumer protection, and the like into accreditation standards.[9]

Accreditation of nursing services is just beginning to receive the same attention from nursing leaders as accreditation of nursing schools.

CONCLUSION

If nursing does not move with deliberate speed to bring about a coordinated system of credentialing, the changes that might well result from what currently exists could be dramatic. With the continued thrust toward reducing costs associated with health care delivery, corporate credentialing might well be viewed as a more appropriate option than those mechanisms currently in use. Since the current political climate seems to be favorable to self-regulation programs, it seems auspicious for all nursing credentialing agencies to come together to build consensus around those issues yet to be resolved.

---

[9] *The Study of Credentialing in Nursing.*

BIBLIOGRAPHY

American Nurses' Association. *A Force for the Nation's Health.* Kansas City, Mo.: ANA 1982.

_____. *The Nursing Practice Act: Suggested State Legislation.* Kansas City, Mo.: ANA, 1980.

_____. *Nursing: A Social Policy Statement.* Kansas City, Mo. ANA, 1980.

_____. *The Study of Credentialing in Nursing: A New Approach.* Kansas City, Mo.: ANA, 1979.

Cole, Eunice R. "Remarks of ANA President." Paper presented at the 53rd Convention of the Hawaii Nurses' Association, Honolulu, Hawaii, November 8, 1984.

LaBar, Clare, "Legal Regulation of Nursing Practice." Paper presented at the Conference on Certification and Assessment of Professional Competence: Toward an Improved Credentialing System in Nursing, San Antonio, Texas, March 1–2, 1984.

Shimberg, Benjamin. "Licensing in the Year 2000." *Issues,* 5 (Summer 1984), pp. 1, 8.

Steel, Jean. "Self-Regulation in the Nursing Profession: The Role of Certification." Paper presented at the Conference on Certification and Assessment of Professional Competence: Toward an Improved Credentialing System in Nursing, San Antonio, Texas, March 1–2, 1984.

New Opportunities in Nursing

THE CORPORATE CONNECTION: MULTIHOSPITAL SYSTEMS REKINDLE COMMITMENT

CONNIE CURRAN, EdD, RN, FAAN
Chairman of Nursing
Montefiore Medical Center
Bronx, New York

Although written early in the 1960s, Bob Dylan's song "The Times They Are A-Changin' " provides a theme that was never more appropriate than it is today—particularly when applied to the health care system. Formerly dominated by a medical orientation, the system is increasingly adopting a health care orientation. Thus, health care institutions have beome very diverse, in terms of both the services they offer and the personnel who provide those services. Not only have the roles of these professionals expanded, but so have their numbers, with the result that many health care agencies are vastly bigger than they were 20 or even 10 years ago. Where once a small center might have cared for a small group of clients, there now often stands a high-rise hospital complex that has merged with other facilities in the same geographic area to provide a wide range of services to a much larger group of clients. Such corporate mergers of hospitals have come to be known as "multihospital systems" (MHSs).

Can bigger mean better? What advantages can be gained from such mergers? Might one disadvantage be that nursing practice in a setting that is part of a large corporation becomes impersonal? A discussion of the nature and history of corporate structures in health care may provide answers to these questions.

WHAT IS A MULTIHOSPITAL SYSTEM?

The multihospital system has developed as part of the trend toward growth in cooperative arrangements among health facilities.[1] According to Ermann and Gabel, both the American Hospital Association and Modern Health Care define multihospital systems as "nonfederal and nonstate hospitals that are either leased, under contract management, legally incorporated, or under the direction of a board that determines the central direction for two or more hospitals."[2] As might be expected from this definition, the interinstitutional arrangements of these systems are varied; in fact, Mason identified seven organizational models, differentiated from one another by the purposes for which the systems were created.[3] A brief description of each model follows.

1. *Formal affiliation.* A close association under a formal agreement, usually for conducting a joint education program; for example, a nursing school affiliated with a hospital for educational programs.

2. *Shared or cooperative services.* A formal or informal agreement to share administrative or clinical services, which can be provided either by a single hospital; by a group of hospitals; or through a separate, taxable, or tax-exempt organization.

3. *Consortia for planning or education.* Voluntary alliances of institutions, usually in the same geographic area, for a specific purpose, most often planning or education.

4. *Contract management.* Total responsibility for management of a health facility is contracted to a separate group for a specified period.

5. *Lease or condominium.* Involves the transfer of property under a contract at a specified rental fee for a specific period, or ownership of shared and unique space in a single facility.

6. *Corporate ownership, separate management.* Assets are owned by a single organization, but management responsibilities are delegated to another party by the owner.

7. *Integrated ownership and management.* Assets are owned and managed by a single entity.

Two basic kinds of organization have evolved: the horizontal and the vertical. A horizontal organization is one that involves sharing, cooperation, coordination, or merger of *like* institutions, whereas a vertical

---

[1] S. Mason, "The Multihospital Movement Defined," *Public Health Reports,* 94, No. 5 (1979), pp. 446–453.

[2] D. Ermann and J. Gabel, "Multihospital Systems, Issues, and Empirical Findings," *Health Affairs,* 3, No. 1 (1984), p. 51.

[3] Mason, "The Multihospital Movement Defined."

organization involves *unlike* institutions. Vertical organizations may include nursing homes, hospices, day care centers, and ambulatory and home health care services.[4]

One out of three hospitals in the United States, accounting for nearly 36 percent of the nation's hospital beds, belongs to a multihospital system, and some experts predict that by 1986, 70 percent of the nation's hospitals will belong to an MHS.[5] In the summer of 1984, two nonprofit hospital systems merged into a 233-unit chain of 45,000 beds, making it the largest multihospital system in the country.[6]

Why do mergers seem to be such an attractive solution to hospitals' management problems? An examination of those problems makes it obvious. Too many hospitals suffer from overbedding, and thus are such poor financial risks that they have difficulty in securing the long-term loans needed for the modernization of equipment and plant that would make them competitive. The advent of diagnosis-related groups (DRGs) has increased the pressure. It has become advantageous for institutions in close physical proximity to collaborate rather than compete, particularly when contending with obsolete buildings and with the continuing need to stay abreast of technology. Analysis of community needs often reveals that the volume of patients justifies one service in the area, not two. Thus, two physically close institutions may fail to get planning permission to build or to acquire new equipment, while a merged organization may have no difficulty in securing approval.

A related problem is that competing facilities may be unable to attract and keep medical staff; once again, formation of an MHS can help, since an attractive, modern facility with a solid volume of admissions is more easily provided by an MHS than by competing hospitals.

HISTORICAL BACKGROUND

How did hospitals come to be in this position in the first place? A review of the historical development of hospitals indicates that their growth patterns have been shaped by their effort to respond to public trends. The 1920s saw rapid growth, due to public acceptance of surgery, laboratory medicine, and radiology. The patient's cost at that time was $10 per day and was considered high. Until this time, 50 percent of all hospitals were proprietary. During the depression of the 1930s, this expansion leveled off. In the 1940s, basic medical research increased because of World War II, and hospitals increased their services to provide research

---

[4] R. MacStravic, "Many Benefits Possible with Vertical System," *Hospitals,* 53, No. 24 (1979), pp. 67–70; and R. Brueck, "Organization and Management of Vertical Systems Face Constraints," *Hospitals,* 55, No. 23 (1981), pp. 65–69.

[5] Ermann and Gabel, "Multihospital Systems."

[6] "Two Non-Profit Hospital Systems Merged into a 233 Unit Chain," *Health Policy Week,* 13, No. 33 (1984).

data and receive research money. In the 1950s, the Hill-Burton Act supported the development of rural hospital systems, which some believe were the precursors of multihospital systems. Although this resulted in an increase in the availability of medical services to rural areas, it was also responsible for an unchecked building spree.

The 1960s witnessed refinements in hospital regulation due to Medicaid and Medicare regulation as well as the development of ancillary health care services. During the Great Society era, federal funds supported increased social services, while medical technology advanced and intensive care units came into great demand. The public expected the latest in technological wonders, regardless of the cost. The unchecked physical growth of hospitals and the runaway inflation rates for medical services laid hospitals open to attack during the efforts at wage and price controls of the 1970s. Hence, the National Planning and Resources Development Act of 1974 was enacted as this country's first step toward systematizing the organization of medical care. The priorities articulated in Section 1502 of Public Law 93–641 mandated:

> 1) The development of multi-institutional systems for coordination or consolidation of institutional health services. 2) The development of multi-institutional arrangements for the sharing of support services necessary to all health service institutions.[7]

QUESTIONS AND PRELIMINARY ANSWERS

Thus, a combination of economic necessity and governmental pressure has made the comparatively new phenomenon of the multihospital system so important in the contemporary health care scene. One might question whether the economic benefit of a merger translates into cheaper service to the client and whether multihospital systems provide more accessible care of higher quality than was possible before the merger. In 1976, Brown and Lewis listed these among the predicted advantages of MHSs; another was the increased economic and political power of multihospital systems.[8] These authors also predicted, however, that increased centralization would lead to disadvantages such as unresponsiveness to local needs on the part of the larger system; intrasystem conflicts that would politicize it; and increased bureaucracy that would drain away some of its economic benefits. On the other hand, a multihospital system might be more effective in raising funds than the constituent institutions were individually. Moreover, the very fact that a merger may

---

[7] H. Zuckerman, "Multi-Institutional Systems: Promise and Performance," *Inquiry*, 16, No. 44 (1979), pp. 291–314.

[8] M. Brown and J. L. Lewis, *Hospital Management Systems: Multiunit Organization and Delivery of Health Care* (Germantown, Md.: Aspen Systems Corp.)

have brought facilities with different functions into a multihospital system might force that system to analyze its mission and role.[9]

In their review of empirical studies of multihospital systems, economists Ermann and Gabel found that the *cost of care* in an MHS is *higher* than it was before merger, particularly for the first few years.[10] This cost increase is evident whether hospital expenses, charges, or revenues are used as the indicator. The increase has been more evident in systems operating for profit than in nonprofit systems. Moreover, there is no difference in the *quality of care* provided by independent and MHS institutions, using qualifications of staff physicians, hospital accreditations, and outcome statistics as indicators of quality. (No data on nurses or nursing care were reported.) Finally, when *accessibility of care* was evaluated there was no difference between independent and MHS facilities, using percentage of Medicare and Medicaid patients as indicators of accessibility.

Some of the predicted advantages have materialized, however. There is greater efficiency in management, and economies of scale in purchasing supplies have become evident. Moreover, MHSs have found that their access to loans has improved because they are considered sounder risks than their constituent institutions had been. Kidder, Peabody and Co. reported that 61 percent of multihospital systems' borrowings were given A+ to AAA ratings in the period from 1978 to 1981, whereas only 18 percent of borrowings from independent hospitals were given these ratings.[11]

Furthermore, not all of the disadvantages felt to be inherent in the MHS have as yet become evident. Centralization of corporate organization, for example, has so far not been experienced as contraining by hospital directors.[12] Moreover, there is no evidence in the literature that multihospital systems are less responsive to local needs than their constitutent institutions had been before merging. Perhaps, however, it is too early to tell what the effects of the MHS may be on the community as perceived by its members.

Nevertheless, intrasystems conflicts have arisen in some MHSs and have caused some mergers to fail. The most frequent source of conflict has been disagreement over the philosophy and mission of the institution, rather than problems of bureaucratic organization.[13]

---

[9] Zuckerman, "Multi-Institutional Systems."

[10] Ermann and Gabel, "Multihospital Systems."

[11] *Ibid.*

[12] S. Kleiner, "Study Finds Corporate Structure Influences Hospital Director's Role," *Hospitals*, 56, No. 10 (1982), pp. 46, 49.

[13] S. Hunter, "Failure Factors in Multi-Institutional Systems Formation," *Health Care Management Review*, 8, No. 2 (1983), pp. 37–49.

IMPLICATIONS FOR NURSING

So far, the consequences of MHSs for practice have not been studied. This work is urgent, however, for without these data, it will be difficult for educators to prepare nursing students to work in these settings. Fortunately, the gap in knowledge will soon be filled because many educators will have joint appointments within multihospital systems. In addition to providing information about changes in practice that can be incorporated into education, the trend toward joint appointments will have other beneficial effects. Nurse educators will find their roles expanding to include more clinical practice, and practitioners will find their roles expanding to include formal teaching responsibilities.

The MHS is a new kind of environment for nurses and one in which they have the opportunity to excel, for they are prepared to contribute to all aspects of its development and functioning. Provision must therefore be made for students to learn about the suprasystem of health care services and its opportunities. Nursing curricula must provide knowledge of the various types of systems, so that students can make decisions about employment and their career advancement within these systems. Courses in the economics of health care managment will be essential to all nurses, and both undergraduate and graduate nursing programs must include content on clinical and managerial aspects of care. The quality of nursing care can be an institution's greatest asset or liability. Expert nursing clinicians contribute to reduced patient complications and decreased length of stay. By providing high-quality, cost-effective patient care, the nurse manager becomes a corporate asset.

For nurses with great ambition, the promise of MHS exists in the corporate power structure. Successful multihospital systems have a clearly established plan for the overall system. These include mission, role, objectives, programs, environment, organizational analysis, demographics, and fiscal data.[14] Appropriately prepared nurses can make important conceptual and practical contributions to such planning. Accordingly, master's and doctoral programs must prepare nurses to manage these diverse new models of health care. Courses in health policy, planning, and finance are essential for participation in corporate decision making. Some nurses already occupy corporate nursing roles—positions unknown before 1976. A 1982 study revealed, however, that only 43 percent of MHSs responding had corporate nurse positions.[15] (Unfortunately, only 47 of the 256 multihospital systems that had been asked to respond did so; thus, these data do not provide an accurate idea of how many nurses actually fill these positions.) Beyers believes that nurses' major contribu-

[14] E. Connors and P. Spaulding, "Multi-Institutional Systems Present Pros and Cons to Planning Process," *Hospitals,* 56, No. 12 (1982), pp. 64, 67, 70.

[15] M. Beyers, "Getting on Top of Organizational Change, Part 3: The Corporate Nurse Executive," *The Journal of Nursing Administration,* 14, No. 12 (1984), pp. 32–37.

tion in the MHS would be the development of means to ensure continuity of care among the health care agencies in the system. This entails that nurses come to look at nursing care in the aggregate, rather than from an institution-specific perspective.

EXAMPLES IN PRACTICE

In 1979, James A. Campbell, president of Chicago's Rush/Presbyterian/St. Lukes Medical Center, predicted that university teaching hospitals "will become the anchors of vertical multi-hospital systems."[16] Rush was the first university hospital in the country to do so. Not all MHSs follow this model, however; Montefiore Medical Center, for example, began as a 26-bed home for chronic invalids, and has expanded to become the largest health care institution in New York City's borough of the Bronx. It has eight diverse sites and employs over 2,400 nurses. Its history includes such innovations in health care and service as the first hospital-based home care program in the country, the first institution staffed entirely by RNs (Loeb Center); a hospice program in Beth Abraham, Montefiore's long-term care facility; and a contractual agreement with New York City to provide health services to Rikers Island prison inmates.

Montefiore Medical Center's mission statement, drafted in 1981, indicates a strong commitment to "educate and encourage the professional development of...health providers, so as to produce professionals of high competence and integrity and with a broad view of health services and their roles in society." This mission is concretely evidenced by Montefiore Medical Center's affiliation with the Albert Einstein College of Medicine as well as by its participation in a collaborative educational effort, also supported by the Robert Wood Johnson Foundation, District 1199 (the hospital workers' union), and Herbert H. Lehman College of the City University of New York, to establish the Health Professions Institute in 1976. Located at Lehman College and designed for students from medicine, nursing, social work, and health services administration, the institute provides opportunities for students from different disciplines to learn to function as a team. As undergraduate students, they study together for two years and are placed in the same clinical agency.

Further evidence of this solid commitment to collaboration with education is provided by the fact that the corporate chair for nursing comes with a professorship at Herbert H. Lehman College. This relationship has led to strengthening of the ties between Montefiore Medical Center and the college; this year, 42 nurse clinicians from Montefiore were

---

[16] Quoted in D. Johnson, "Universitites Will Anchor Vertical Systems," *Modern Healthcare,* 9, No. 12 (1979), pp. 50, 53–54.

granted clinical associate titles at Lehman. These clinicians will serve as role models for undergraduate and graduate students at the college as well as serving as guest lecturers and on college committees.

Montefiore's strong commitment to education is demonstrated through its sabbatical leave policy. The sabbatical has long been a tradition in education and is now catching on in business. Montefiore is the first institution of its kind in the country to offer paid sabbatical leave for nurses.

OTHER BENEFITS

Nurses obviously stand to gain from the solid commitment to education that a corporate institution can offer, but this is only one of the possible benefits. The corporate structure of a vertical MHS lends itself far more readily to the creation of a clinical career ladder than a single institution can; opportunities for professional networking are much increased; and participation in corporatewide committees that build policy for the whole system can provide nurses with power and visibility.

At Montefiore Medical Center, for example, a corporatewide clinical ladder committee was formed and charged with identifying the career goals and interests of nurses. This served as a basis to propose opportunities for advancement and for moving from one area of concentration to another, including the ability to transfer from one site to another without losing seniority or benefits.

Nurses at Montefiore Medical Center have their own corporatewide newsletter to increase communication and collaboration. The editorial board meets monthly to decide topics and to coordinate site correspondents' news items. Furthermore, Montefiore nurses have the opportunity to be active on many corporatewide committees comprising staff nurses from all levels and from all sites, such as the committees for sabbaticals, continuing education, and professional standards. The nurse recognition committee, which used to be ad hoc, is now a standing committee charged with establishing guidelines for offering the sabbatical that will be effective systemwide.

CONCLUSION

The effects of the MHS on nursing practice are not yet obvious, so there can be no definite answer to the question of whether such systems make nursing practice more impersonal than it was formerly. Impersonal behavior toward clients may perhaps be preventable, if nurses' own needs for education, career advancement, and recognition can be met. In the contemporary MHS, this is possible as never before; as the experience of Montefiore Medical Center reveals, personal commitment to education and delivery of care is rekindled by the corporate connection.

It creates a power structure for nurses by virtue of their numbers and impact on the health care system that previously did not exist. It creates the opportunity for the development of personal approaches to nursing care and for innovations in practice, education, and research. And, finally, it creates avenues for recognition, advancement, and professional growth.

MARKETING CONTINUING EDUCATION PROGRAMS IN A CLIMATE OF COST CONTAINMENT

LAWRENCE LITWACK, EdD
Chairman, Department of Counseling Psychology,
Rehabilitation, and Special Education
Northeastern University
Boston, Massachussetts

If one were to examine carefully current materials such as the Chronicle of Higher Education, professional journals, and annual reports of health care and educational institutions, it would become quickly and readily apparent that there is a pervading concern about budget reductions and cost containment. In such a financial climate, administrators in all sectors have been seeking ways to reduce expenses and increase income.

Among the items being looked at most closely are the cost of continuing eduation and professional development programs as well as the potential for such programs to generate income. This paper will explore current issues and marketing strategies for continuing education.

BACKGROUND

Definition of Continuing Education

If one were to define continuing education, it would seem desirable to use generally accepted terminology and standards. The Board of Directors of the National League for Nursing approved the following as part of a longer position paper on continuing education:

> Continuing education is a personal evaluative educational experience, objectively planned for individual growth and achievement

153

of knowledge and skills beyond the basic preparation for a profession or occupation. Continuing education is understood to include in-service education but to exclude orientation or on-the-job training considered to be basic preparation for a specific position.[1]

The Council on the Continuing Education Unit defined continuing education as:

> formal education programs/activities for professional development and training, or for credentialing, for which academic credit is not awarded, or of personal interest to the learner, for which academic credit is not awarded.[2]

Regarding the purpose of continuing education, the Council notes:

> A generally accepted purpose of continuing education programs/activities is to help maintain, expand, and improve individual knowledge, skills (performance), and attitude and, by so doing, equally meet the improvement and advancement of individuals, professions, and organizations.[3]

The criteria used as a recognized national standard follow guidelines developed by the National Task Force on the Continuing Education Unit, which award one unit for each ten hours of actual contact in an organized continuing education experience under responsible sponsorship, capable direction, and qualified instruction.[4] These guidelines include elements such as spelled-out, specific, measurable, and attainable objectives, carefully planned programs utilizing principles of adult learning, and the inclusion of specific evaluative criteria and procedures.

Mandatory Continuing Education

An area that has the potential for great impact on the provision of continuing education is the issue of mandatory continuing education. As of 1983, 12 states mandated continuing education for all registered nurses (California, Colorado, Florida, Iowa, Kansas, Kentucky, Massachusetts, Minnesota, Nebraska, Nevada, New Mexico, and South

[1] Executive Committee of the Board of Directors, "Position Statement on NLN's Role in Continuing Education in Nursing" (New York: National League for Nursing, May 1978).

[2] *Principles of Good Practice in Continuing Education,* Report of the CCEU Project to Develop Standards and Criteria for Good Practice in Continuing Education (Silver Spring, Md.: Council on the Continuing Education Unit, April 1984), p. 7.

[3] *Ibid.,* p. 3.

[4] National Task Force on the Continuing Education Unit, *The Continuing Education Unit: Criteria and Guidelines* (Washington, D.C.: National University Extension Association, 1984).

Dakota).[5] Five other states mandate continuing education for nurse practitioners (Alaska, Idaho, Mississippi, New Hampshire, and Oregon).
Three additional states have passed enabling legislation (Louisiana,
Michigan, Washington). For licensed practical nurses, the picture is
similar to that for registered nurses; all of the states mentioned, except
for Minnesota and South Dakota, plus Virginia mandate continuing
education for LPNs.

An important element that must be considered in any discussion of
mandatory continuing education is how that is defined. Examining the
various statutes, one finds that the definition of valid subject matter for
continuing education varies from state to state. For example, California
regulations indicate that

> Course content must be related to scientific knowledge or technical
> skills required for the practice of nursing, or be related to direct
> or indirect patient care.... Courses which deal with self-
> improvement, changes in attitude or financial gain, or [those]
> designed for lay people are unacceptable for license renewal.[6]

New Hampshire regulations define continuing education as that which
"is relevant to the clinical area of the nurse. The content must be such
that it increases the knowledge and skill of the ARNP (Advanced
Registered Nurse Practitioner) in the area of specialty. Attendance at
inservice programs does not meet the C.E. requirements for the
ARNP."[7]

Producers of Continuing Education

Legal mandate is just one of several reasons for the provision of continuing education. A second major reason is to improve professional
practice in order to better meet the health needs of the community. A
third reason is as a possible aid to student recruitment. If educational
institutions provide continuing education opportunities for nurses, some
of them may develop an interest in enrolling in formal advanced degree
programs. A fourth reason is to produce revenue to support other institutional or agency programs that may be important, but not cost-
effective. A fifth reason, exemplified by the entrepreneurship of private
groups or individuals, is to produce revenue for profit. A final reason
for the provision of programs is to meet specific needs expressed by a
variety of specialty groups.

---

[5] Christopher Wellisa, "Professionals Debate Value of Brush-Ups," in "The Summer Survey of
Education," *New York Times,* August 22, 1982, Sec. 12, p. 12; and "CE Now Required for
Relicensure in 16 States," *American Journal of Nursing,* 82 (November 1982), pp. 1668, 1675.

[6] Quoted in "CE Now Required for Relicensure in 16 States," p. 1668.

[7] Quoted in *Ibid.*

With these reasons in mind, it is easy to understand the range of producers of continuing education program opportunities. Within educational institutions, we see programs provided by specific academic units on a decentralized basis or by a centralized department or division of continuing education in cooperation with the appropriate academic unit. Among professional associations, programs are provided on the national level by groups such as NLN, American Nurses' Association, American Hospital Association, American Public Health Association, and National Association for Practical Nurse Education and Service; on the regional level by groups such as the Midwest Alliance in Nursing and the NLN regional assemblies; on the state level by groups such as NLN constituent leagues or state nursing associations; and on the local level by groups such as district nurse associations. The third major provider groups come from a variety of profit-making, private organizations that offer packaged programs. It is important to note that the provider of the continuing education program is not necessarily the granter of the continuing education unit.

Audience for Programs

Obviously, the audience for continuing education programs must be considered in planning program offerings. In 1982, NLN commissioned Arthur D. Little to do a study on the markets for NLN products and services in nursing education and nursing service. The study was done in two phases. Phase 1 involved individual and group interviews with NLN staff members and volunteers, individuals in 50 educational and service organizations, and groups of nursing administrators and faculty. Phase 2 involved a telephone survey of nurse educators and nurse administrators from all levels of nursing education and sites of nursing service. As a result of the in-depth interviews, the study identified, in order of priority, continuing education topics of significant interest for particular groups. These are shown in Table 1.

The Arthur D. Little study provides some useful information. However, it was primarily targeted at nursing education and nursing service. Several other target groups are potential recipients of continuing education programs.

One of these is composed of consumers of health services. This, of course, would include members of populations at risk, such as the poor, elderly, and disabled. However, if we are equally committed to promoting wellness and preventing illness, then programs can be provided for the community at large dealing with a variety of health-related issues.

A second target group would be made up of members of allied health provider groups. This might include nursing home administrators (as of 1982, 42 states mandate continuing education for them), physicians (for whom 20 states mandate continuing education), and social workers (for whom 15 states mandate continuing education). Other groups, such

Table 1. Identified Continuing Education Topics in Nursing Education and Nursing Service, in Order of Priority

Level or area	Category	CE Topic
Nursing Education		
Baccalaureate	Management	Leadership skills
		Basic management
	Clinical	Pharmacology
	Other	Computers/programming
		Teaching strategies
		Telecommunications
Diploma	Management	Basic management
		Finance and budgeting
	Clinical	Critical care nursing
		Hyperalimentation
	Other	Teaching strategies
		Telecommunications
		Computers/programming
Associate degree	Management	Leadership skills
		Basic management
	Clinical	Pharmacology
		Pediatrics
		Obstetrics/gynecology
		Cardiovascular/pulmonary nursing
	Other	Computers/programming
		Teaching strategies
		Telecommunications
Practical nursing	Management	Leadership skills
		Time management
	Clinical	Pharmacology
		Pediatrics
		Obstetrics/gynecology
	Other	Computers/programming
		Teaching strategies
		Telecommunications
Nursing Service		
Hospitals	Management	Leadership skills
		Basic management
		Finance and budgeting
	Clinical	Pharmacology
		Cardiovascular/pulmonary nursing

Table 1, continued

Level or area	Category	CE Topic
	Other	Obstetrics/gynecology
		Critical care
		Intensive care
		Teaching strategies
		Computers/programming
		Telecommunications
Long-term care	Management	Leadership skills
		Basic management
		Finance and budgeting
	Clinical	Geriatric care
	Other	Computers/programming
		Teaching strategies
Home/community health	Management	Leadership skills
		Time management
		Personnel
	Clinical	Geriatric care
		Cardiovascular/pulmonary nursing
		Hyperalimentation
		Oncology
		IV therapy
	Other	Computers/programming
		Teaching strategies

as medical technicians, respiratory technicians, emergency medical technicians, physicians' assistants, and the like might also be included, since many share common concerns.

A third target group can be found in single-purpose, special interest health-related groups such as ostomy groups, Reach for Recovery, Alcoholics Anonymous, Narcotics Anonymous, Alateen, Al-Anon, and cancer societies. Frequently, members of such groups have great interest in new developments in prevention or treatment in a particular area. By broadening the base of potential recipients of continuing education, it may be possible to widen the range and frequency of program offerings.

MARKETING STRATEGIES

With this background in mind, it is time to turn to some specific marketing strategies. To do a better job of providing a wide range of continuing education programs, there are a variety of techniques that can be used and steps that can be taken to increase the likelihood of programs' success. The following are suggested as ways of facilitating the conception and development of programs.

Needs Assessment

What is and is not currently being provided in the geographic region served by the sponsoring organization? How accessible are existing programs in terms of time, cost, location, and the like? The results of such an assessment will help avoid direct competition with existing programs and will help identify unmet needs.

Planning

Include representatives from the proposed target audience as members of the planning committee. Check any existing coordinating calendars to avoid direct scheduling conflicts. If no such master calendar exists, consider serving as the spearhead to start one, since all groups would benefit.

Learn from Others

Whenever possible, utilize successful concepts applied elsewhere. Look at evaluations of previous programs and speakers, including reasons for failures or cancellations of programs.

Cosponsorship

Several departments or programs within an institution or various professional groups, such as nurses and social workers, may cosponsor programs. Cosponsorship may be undertaken with other groups that mandate or recommend continuing education, particularly in cross-discipline areas that share common concerns such as stress management, burnout, leadership, computers, and the like. It may be done with allied groups such as the American Association of Retired Persons, Gray Panthers, and ostomy groups. Cosponsorship may also be undertaken among local, regional, or national groups—for example NLN, regional assemblies, constituent leagues, councils, and educational institutions. The latter approach is being done more within the league's structure.

Media

With the increased cost of travel, greater attention needs to be given to the possibility of media approaches. These include the use of techniques such as teleconferences; videotapes of national speakers with local reactors; audio- or videotaping programs for later use or resale; and packaged programs, programmed instruction, and modular learning packages.

Cost Containment

Location. Look for donated space instead of hotels—in schools, hospitals, and the like. The cost is usually minimal or nonexistent.

Equipment. Use only what is necessary for the group's size. Try to borrow equipment such as projectors.

Materials. Prepare only what is necessary. Duplicate materials in advance. If materials are extensive, consider packaging them for sale to participants.

Meals and Refreshments. If food is easily available elsewhere within an appropriate time frame, its provision can be reduced or eliminated.

Mailing. Costs of mailings may be shared with sponsoring groups or donated by an institution or community group.

Transportation. Whenever possible, bring programs to participants rather than participants to programs.

Publicity

1. Publicize the program well in advance—two to three months minimum beforehand. Watch deadlines for continuing education approval from other groups, if it is desired, to broaden the potential audience.

2. Have clearly stated program title, objectives, and outcomes.

3. Clearly indicate sponsoring group or groups.

4. Get mailing lists from all cosponsors.

5. List the program in media calendars—on radio, on television, in newspapers, and so forth.

6. Target specific groups that are potentially interested in the topic being presented.

7. Send an announcement to all participants in previous programs.

8. Clearly identify the costs of the program, including any special arrangements for retirees, students, non-group members, or bulk registrations.

Quality Control

Program evaluation by participants must be built into the program's time frame. If the program is not top quality or cannot be provided as advertised, do not schedule it or, if at all possible, cancel the program rather than offer something of inferior quality that will jeopardize future program offerings.

CEUs and Registrants' Records

Cost of continuing education units (CEUs) and registrants' records must be carefully figured, including the ease and convenience of both storage and retrieval upon individuals' request.

SUMMARY

If we hope to expand continuing education programming, then we will need to develop a much greater variety of program designs and formats and to develop a specific identity of our own rather than attempt to directly compete with others. We will also need greater involvement of speakers and program participants in program planning and follow-up activities. Incorporation of the ideas expressed in this paper will greatly enhance program offerings and increase partnerships among a variety of constituent groups. Through cooperation can come quality and service; through competition can come mediocrity and unmet needs.

INTERNATIONAL NURSING EDUCATION

SISTER ROSEMARY DONLEY, PhD, RN
Dean of Nursing
Catholic University of America
and
SISTER MARY JEAN FLAHERTY, PhD, RN
Chairperson, Nursing of the Developing Family
Catholic University of America
Washington, D.C.

This essay will discuss international education from three perspectives: the education of international nurses in American colleges and universities; the roles that American nurses play around the world as educators, practitioners, consultants and participants in study tours; and the influence of American nursing literature on the education of international nurses.

Several assumptions, which are based on the experience of the authors, guide the discussion:

1. The number of international nursing students enrolled in American schools will increase.

2. As nurses expand their world views, overseas travel and professional exchange will become attractive ways to vacation and visit other health care systems. In the future, more nurse educators and practitioners will accept overseas assignments.

3. English is the language of high technology, medicine, and nursing.

These assumptions will each be discussed in turn.

INTERNATIONAL STUDENTS

The assumption that there will be an increasing number of international students reflects a changing American demography as well as a demand for nurses generated by the international development of high technology health care. American colleges, especially in the Northeast, are looking overseas to fill their classrooms. Will international recruitment affect education in general and nursing in particular?

Most international students experience some difficulty in American classrooms. The informal atmosphere, the values assigned to student participation and discussion, and the use of multiple choice tests may overwhelm bright students. American pedagogy is especially difficult for students whose earlier education espoused respect for the authority and wisdom of teachers and encouraged memorization and analysis of texts. In nursing, clinical education is integral to the discipline. Communication is central to the establishment of nurse-patient relationships, and language is the tool of assessment and care. Understanding human responses to illness and health demands a grasp of dominant values and norms. Nursing students confront a foreign culture in ways unknown to their countrymen and women who major in engineering, music, or arts and sciences.

Because of the nature of the program of study in the nursing major, competency in language is a criterion to be weighed in admission decisions. Scores on the Test of English as a Foreign Language (TOEFL), which may serve as a predictor of success for the arts and sciences faculty, may not adequately guide decisions about nursing students. Licensed nurses who come to America to earn degrees face a series of special examinations or rites of passage. Not only must these nurse demonstrate visa clearances; certificates of good health; academic records that indicate competence; appropriate scores on the TOEFL; evidence that they read, speak, and understand English; and academic and personal solvency, but they are also asked to obtain a certificate from the Commission on Graduates of Foreign Nursing Schools (COGFNS). In some jurisdictions, licensed international nurses must write the National Council Licensure Examination for Registered Nurses (NCLEX) before they can participate in anything other than traditional undergraduate supervised practice in their clinical studies. These special requirements test the perseverance as well as the competence of international nurses and highlight the importance that should be given to decisions to admit international students to U.S. schools of nursing.

The decision to attend a particular school is influenced by the catalog and by familiarity with faculty who publish in journals available to international students and facuty. Leone reports that students look for the word "international" in catalogs and read the first letter from the school to which they have applied with great care.[1] She urges that written information be descriptive of the program of study and present requirements as achievable goals rather than barriers.

When the international student matriculates, it becomes obvious to faculty that educational and scholarly values are formed within cultures. By international standards, America has a limited tradition of scholarship. International students are surprised that most of their classmates and teachers speak one language and accept high school and college education as normative behavior. In most countries of the world, places in college-preparatory high schools and first-rate universities are reserved for those who pass competitive examinations or come from upper-class families. Consequently, most international students ascribe status to the student role and consider it to be a position of privilege. They are eager and willing to invest energy and time in their academic work and are often bewildered by the cavalier attitudes of American students who merely play at the education enterprise.

Although most international students hold high standards of scholarship, their values are different. For example, the American definition of plagiarism seems strange to students who memorize, quote, and appropriate the texts and the words of their teachers. Another difference becomes evident when international students engage in discussions or write term papers. The simple linear relationship that Americans see between ideas A and B may be unclear to students trained in different traditions of logic. They may see a relationship between ideas A and C, because it is more consonant with their cognitive structures. Because of these differences, evaluation of the written work of international students requires sensitivity to logic, academic standards, and the use of language.

The presence of international students on campus also creates subtle changes in the learning environment of American students—changes that are frequently overlooked in discussions of international education. Although academic requirements remain the same for both groups of students, the international student brings a different perspective to clinical experiences and classroom discussions. For many Americans, the opportunity to study with international students is their first exposure to foreign cultures. American students hear about new value systems, different definitions of health and illness, unique priorities in the allocation of resources, and health care systems that bear little resemblance to familiar patterns. The richness of the exchange of ideas between American and international students adds a dimension of understanding, tolerance, and flexibility.

A variation on this theme is reported by Schenk in a description of

[1] L. P. Leone, "Orienting Nurses from Other Countries to Graduate Education in the United States," *Journal of Nursing Education*, 21, No. 7 (1982), pp. 45–47.

American nursing students studying in England.[2] She reports that the students' education was enriched by their ability to compare the American system of health care with the model operating in Great Britain. Amin describes similar values in a cross-cultural, three-week study-travel course that brings American nursing students to Egypt and Israel.[3]

The appearance of international nurses in American classrooms is evidence that dramatic changes are operative not only in first-world countries, but in third- and fourth-world societies as well. The development of tertiary care centers in the OPEC nations and the existence of CAT scanners in Indonesia are illustrations of the impact of change on health beliefs and practices. As third-world countries import high technology medicine, they need nurses who can manage the machinery, negotiate with physicians trained in the West, and give intensive care to patients. The enrollment of nurses from third-world countries in critical care courses or degree programs highlights the tension created when technology runs ahead of personnel development. Ironically, these nurses come to study in a country that is reevaluating its commitment to high technology health care and struggling with the escalating health costs and ethical dilemmas that accompany tertiary care.

It is obvious from this discussion that international students of nursing require unique support from faculty and institution. Although the special needs of international students may diminish over time, colleges that admit international students have a continuing responsibility to assist them with relocation and culture shock, as well as to arrange their programs of study. Failure to provide sufficient help for international students produces anguish and may lead to academic failure, illness, depression, or the need to return home. Tien gives meaning to this statement by poignantly describing her distress at failing a graduate preliminary examination because of "poor synthesizing ability."[4] Tien reported feeling betrayed, insulted, and angry. Her plight was mitigated by a faculty member in mental health nursing. This teacher helped her understand what the examining committee meant by their comments and enabled her to succeed. The strategies that were developed included independent study, additional course work, therapy, and the employment of a tutor who helped Tien present herself in "an American way."

U.S. NURSES ABROAD

Our second assumption is that more American nurses will go abroad

[2] K. Schenk, "Nursing Abroad in an Undergraduate Program," *International Nursing Review*, 27, No. 4 (1980), pp. 108–109.

[3] Afaf El-Gazzar Amin, "Cross-Cultural Awareness: A Nursing Imperative," *International Nursing Review*, 31, No. 1 (1984), pp. 9–10.

[4] J. Tien, "Surviving Graduate Nursing Programs in the United States—A Personal Account of an Asian-American Student," *Journal of Nursing Education*, 21, No. 7, pp. 42–44.

to teach, administer, consult, or visit other health care systems. Many nurses will be attracted to the world market by the exportation of high technology medicine. As ministries of health debate how they will spend their health dollars, specialist physicians trained in the United States collaborate with international developers in building tertiary health care systems. Nurses in these countries, oriented by education to midwifery, community nursing, and primary care, are out of place in the intensive care units. The deficit in prepared nurses creates a void that is filled by nurses from other countries. For example, Bahrain, a country in the Arabian Gulf, reported 1,115 budgeted nursing positions in 1983.[5] National nurses filled only 22 percent of the posts. Expatriates, mainly from Iran, India, Pakistan, Korea, and the Philippines, provided the majority of the nursing force.

The transition from primary care to high technology health systems is painful and difficult. The ability of some countries to develop a cadre of educated nurses is related to the image of nursing as a career option for women.[6] In many developing countries, basic education in nursing occurs at the end of junior high school. It is difficult to provide advanced training and education to people who lack basic education in science. Physicians, who frequently provide in-service programs to upgrade the education of practicing nurses, become impatient with disparities between medical initiation and management of high technology regimens and the nursing staff's ability to provide comparable levels of nursing care.

The desire to create an "instant nurse force" to care for very sick patients has produced several scenarios. One common practice is to recruit American nurses to offer short-term training programs for traditionally prepared nationals. This "Band-Aid" preparation of tertiary care nurses creates dissonance among nurses and teachers and is usually short-lived. When this practice is abandoned, a multinational nurse force is recruited to staff intensive care units. This solution is so firmly established in several Middle Eastern countries that these governments advertise in American nursing journals for critical care nurses and nurse faculty. A long-range outcome of the failure of short-term educational programs is a reevaluation of traditional patterns of educating nurses.

Restructuring nursing education involves political decisions. Some of the important factors, as outlined by Masson, are selection of a curriculum model (English, French, or American); evaluation of the role of physicians; determination of the influence of the government as authority shifts from ministries of health (hospital-based) to ministries of education (university-based); and development of faculty and

[5] N. M. Kronfal and F. Affara, "Nursing Education in the Arabian Gulf: The Bahrain Model," *International Journal of Nursing Studies,* 19, No. 2 (1982), pp. 89–98.

[6] A. Meleis and S. Hanson, "Oil Rich, Nurse Poor: The Nursing Crisis in the Persian Gulf," *Nursing Outlook,* 28, No. 4 (1980), pp. 238–243.

resources.[7] If the country chooses a university system of education, students are sent to study abroad and American nurse educators are invited to consult, direct, or teach in programs of nursing. American educators, seasoned by the difficulty within their own community in implementing baccalaureate education, are overwhelmed by the effects of a governmental mandate on educational systems. However, they soon discover that an executive or legislative imperative does not create a faculty, a library, a curriculum, clinical mentors, or a student body prepared to study nursing science. These resources require the combined efforts of nurse educators and national nursing leaders. Successful programs characteristically receive government and medical endorsement.

It is anticipated that both short- and long-range strategies to educate international nurses will be utilized in the future. However, as more national nurses are educated in the United States or in baccalaureate and graduate programs within their own countries, short-term educational programs will assume less importance as a personnel development strategy.

ENGLISH AS THE LANGUAGE OF NURSING

The third assumption of this paper identifies the literature as a tool of cultural exchange. English is the language of medicine and nursing. The authors' experience as leaders of study tours in Taiwan, Korea, the Philippines, Hong Kong, Spain, Kenya, and China and as teachers of students from 25 countries supports our assumption that American literature influences the conceptualization of nursing around the world. Work with the World Health Organization in Southeast Asia reinforces the belief that professional literature exercises a profound impact on nursing practice in distant parts of the world. It is impressive to be asked about the nursing process in a remote health center in a mountain jungle area. Gosnell also observed this phenomenon in Papua, New Guinea.[8]

In classrooms of the world where nursing is taught in a second language, English is the language of instruction. When instruction occurs in the primary language, nursing students study American texts and journals and listen as their teachers discuss nursing practice as it is described in American literature.

The scarcity of library resources can hamper students' use of national or world literature. Masson notes that the expense of importing nursing literature causes faculty to restrict students' access to books and

[7] V. Masson, "International Collaboration in Nursing Education: The People to People Approach," *Journal of Nursing Education*, 19, No. 5 (1980), pp. 48-54.

[8] D. Gosnell, "Introducing the Nursing Process in Papua, New Guinea," *International Nursing Review*, 29, No. 6 (1981), pp. 108-109, 115.

journals.⁹ The traditional practice of reading from notes, a well-established method of education, also encourages national teachers to keep articles and textual material for the development of their lectures. American nurses can compare their personal libraries to the libraries in schools of nursing around the world.

The development of university-based systems of nursing education will be reflected in the libraries of the world. American nurses will play increasingly influential roles in the world as American literature is imported. This trend is particularly interesting because most American authors do not realize that they are writing for an international community. It is usually publishers who tell authors that their books have been translated into Spanish or Japanese. Another sign of the parochial orientation of American authors is the relative absence of international citations in the reviews of literature that accompany their writings. As American nurses have more contact with international students here and abroad, they will develop a more cosmopolitan orientation in their work.

Social theorists suggest that ours is a global culture. It is not surprising, therefore, that international exchange is the experience of Americans. What is remarkable is the influence that American nurses have on education and practice around the world. This influence can only be extended as more students from other countries study and practice under the aegis of American nurses. The tools of cultural exchange are the curriculum, the literature, and—perhaps the oldest technique of all—the student-teacher relationship.

One of the gifts that has been given to American nurse educators is the opportunity to influence world health. They do this by teaching the next generation of international nurses and their teachers to identify and study human phenomena and to change social structures, so that health for all by the year 2000 will be an action plan as well as a goal.¹⁰

⁹ Masson, "International Collaboration in Nursing Education."

¹⁰ D. Krebs, "ICN's Program on Nursing in Primary Health Care: Present and Future. *International Nursing Review*, 29, No. 6 (1982), pp. 167–168.

PREPARING CLINICAL SPECIALISTS FOR PROSPECTIVE PAYMENT

LUCILLE A. JOEL, EdD, FAAN
Professor and Director for Clinical Affairs
Director, Teaching Nursing Home Project
Rutgers University College of Nursing
Newark, New Jersey

Since the introduction of the clinical nurse specialist role, debate has prevailed over the knowledge, skills, and activities basic to practice and the organizational structure that best facilitates execution of this role. These issues have risen to new prominence in a climate of economic constraint. A natural reaction to the rising cost of health care has been to challenge the value of services and providers of care. Highly qualified and skilled caretakers will be especially scrutinized because of their greater financial compensation. Inability to demonstrate a contribution to organizational fiscal integrity will force the substitution of less skilled and consequently less costly options. This is the challenge clinical specialists face.

This paper will present a brief analysis of the dynamics responsible for changes in health care as well as predictions of the nature of those changes. The clinical nurse specialist, used appropriately, can guide the profession to a position of power in times that may often seem devoid of opportunity.

BEFORE AND AFTER PROSPECTIVE PAYMENT

The introduction of Medicare prospective pricing added momentum to events that had already begun to reshape the health care delivery system. The singular most influential dynamic in changing patterns of health care has been a process called "cost shifting."

For many years prior to prospective payment, Medicare patients and Medicaid patients in many states were reimbursed on the basis of cost. These patients paid less for their hospital care than individuals insured

by private sector companies. The government negotiated rates based
on the cost of services, as opposed to the common practice of inflating
certain costs to charge amounts that cross-subsidized departments or
services that were not cost efficient. The next step toward reducing
government's investment in health care, and specifically acute care, was
the move from "cost" to "case mix" reimbursement, setting upper limits
for each patient based on clinical characteristics associated with resource
consumption. This is the diagnosis-related group (DRG) methodology.
A cost-efficient hospital will probably fare better financially under DRGs
than under cost reimbursement. Cost reimbursement limited a hospital
to receiving exactly what service cost it, with no provisions for more
effective care or more efficient management. Even though some financial gains may be possible under DRGs, for the most part Medicare
and Medicaid patients do not share equally in hospital expenses. An
additional financial liability for hospitals is created by the group we have
come to label "bad debt" or "uncompensated care." These are the individuals who fall through the safety net that Medicare and Medicaid
provided adequately in the past. This population is no longer the poor
but is now most notably the unemployed who are not at the welfare level
and those in transition between jobs—people who are financially
devastated if struck by illness.

Both the deficit created by Medicare and Medicaid patients and the
cost of uncompensated care are shifted to private sector insurers and
those few individuals who continue to pay out of pocket. By the end
of 1984, $8.3 billion will have been "cost shifted" to the private sector.[1]
The net result has been increased premiums. Group coverage originating
in the workplace and included in part or whole as an employee benefit
insures 160 million Americans. This fact has promoted business and
industry to include provisions in health care policies that aim to reshape
utilization practices. Incentives discourage the use of more costly settings
and providers. A limitation of reimbursement for a preoperative hospital
stay to 24 hours for elective surgery is common, so that patients are forced
to have preoperative testing done on an ambulatory basis. Many plans
offer 100 percent coverage for services provided in freestanding ambulatory care settings but require a copayment or deductible if the same
care is received in a hospital emergency room or outpatient clinic.
Hospital-based facilities are more costly because of the shared burden
of overhead and technology. In some plans, access to medical specialists
is limited and is only reimbursed after referral from a primary care provider. One large industry has begun to establish personal funds for each
employee. The personal fund might start, hypothetically, at a level of
$300 annually and can be used for any health-related needs—services

[1] *Health Care Cost Containment: A Guide for New Jersey Employers* (Trenton: New Jersey Business and
Industry Association, July 1984).

that are not covered or that employees pay out of pocket. The personal fund may be increased by $200 if the employee has dependent coverage, and the health care of those dependents becomes the responsibility of a spouse employed in another company. The employee's policy could then be reduced to single-person coverage. The plan could again be increased by $200 if the individual has a working spouse who can guarantee full family coverage. The employee would then waive all rights to this benefit through his or her primary employer. In most instances, the amount that has not been used at the end of the year reverts either fully or partially to the employee as a reward for prudent buying practices.

We are observing a cause and effect that is very American in character. Once government begins to intrude into our lives, private enterprise retaliates with initiatives that address the ultimate goal with added creativity and aggressiveness. To keep the heavy hand of government out of their lives, Americans will ''hold the line'' on health care costs. Health care utilization practices will shift dramatically from hospitals to a community-based freestanding organizational context and to an emphasis on self-care and natural support systems.

Insurance provisions that are recast in a new model will shrink hospital use. To have any true economic effect, hospitals themselves will have to shrink and cater to those who truly need residential care. The fiscal integrity of hospitals is contingent on a complex case mix, decreased length of stay, and increased volume and maximum occupancy rates. Every bed will be filled, but there are going to be less beds. Patients will be admitted and discharged rapidly, and every case, whether simple or complex, will be viewed with an eye to further decreasing length of stay. Patients will come to the hospital for one of two things: surgery or nursing. There is not much else that cannot be handled in the community. If patients do not come to the hospital for nursing, they stay for nursing. They stay for education, counseling, or restoration of their self-care abilities or because community or family supports are inadequate. Inpatients will become predominately the chronically ill and aged—populations who have traditionally needed intensive nursing services.

FINANCIAL SURVIVAL THROUGH CLINICAL SPECIALIZATION

The predicted nature of hospitalized patients and the expected qualifications for hospitals' economic survival will create a unique opportunity for nursing to emerge as an economic force in hospitals. State-of-the-art nursing can significantly affect length of stay, avoid or minimize complications, and ensure documentation of complications of a borderline clinical nature. Complications may only increase trim points one to two days but may have a much more profound toll on use of resources. Generation of revenue through incentives is clearly probable. Nursing can change the usual roles of professional health care providers and their utilization practices and begin to force internal budget shifts. Sophisticated nursing observations can affect physician's ordering practices. It is time to reassess earlier decisions to allow some of our historic responsibilities to be assumed by other provider groups. Decisions on the need for respiratory therapists for oxygen and inhalation treatments, physical therapists for ambulation, transfer, and range of motion, and so on have to be reconsidered in terms of cost and efficacy. Thus, nursing can directly and visibly contribute to the economic survival of hospitals by creating incentives and turning cases that have been losers into winners. Nursing's financial survival in those settings will also be contingent on digging into the budgets of other departments and petitioning for budget increases based on the rise in nursing intensity.

The clinical gains detailed here require state-of-the-art nursing at the bedside. In the 1980s, "state-of-the-art" is beyond the grasp of the entry-level practitioner and is definitely the province of the clinical specialist. Such statements bring us full circle to a discussion of the organizational structure that will get care of this sophistication to the patient. Controversy focuses on the issues of power versus powerlessness and influence versus authority. Who is the clinical nurse specialist accountable to, and for what? What is the clinical specialist's scope of authority, if any? The answers lie in the knowledge and skill basic to the role, which in turn defines its uniqueness. Even that response is less than clear. The wise urge us to tolerate ambiguity and avoid the pitfalls of overly constraining role definitions. Conversely, many clinical nurse specialists in the front lines strain to clarify their role and seek security through delimiting job descriptions and the protective mantle of regulatory boards. In fact, legislative advocacy in 40 states has resulted in the regulatory protection of titles for advanced practice. Titles such as "nurse clinician," "clinical nurse specialist," "nurse practitioner," "adult nurse practitioner," "diabetic nurse," and so on are controlled by law.[2] Such precipitous activity is based on the fantasy that some kind of generic security is possible, instead of on the healthier attitude that knowledge and demonstrated impact are power.

A search for consensus on effective and efficient utilization models should begin with an analysis of the current realities of practice, tempered by the prevailing educational models. The resulting judgments on appropriate and necessary function should facilitate decisions on administrative control and authority, which are surrounded by controversy. The changing nature of the delivery system has already been established.

The educational preparation of the clinical nurse specialist provides

[2] Francis I. Waddle, "Legal Regulation of Nursing Practice" (Kansas City, Mo.: American Nurses' Association, September 1981) (mimeographed).

maximum flexibility for the workplace. The clinical nurse specialist can well be identified as a generalist in role. Competencies of the teacher, the manager, the direct caregiver, the researcher, and the consultant are all included in the preparation for the role. Which role components emerge as central in a particular employment situation will be determined by organizational need. Questions of staff or line use of specialists are also resolved in the workplace. The clearest direction for the use of the clinical nurse specialist comes from an analysis of where nursing in an institution is at a given point in time. The nature of nursing personnel at the bedside is the determining factor. If a professional nurse is at the bedside, more distance and personal responsibility may be justified in the staff relationship. Professionals value the fact that within any field of work there are specialists. Professionals accept that there is much they do not know and that there is always a more scientific answer, an added dimension to a situation that escapes them because they do not have the knowledge. Professionals value consultation from people who know more, have done more, and have been prepared at a higher level. They weigh carefully recommendations obtained through consultation, incorporate them into their practice, and apply them long enough to evaluate their benefit. With that type of person at the bedside, you do not need to carry a big stick. In this instance, clinical control is through influence. The clinical specialist has no legitimate authority, but relies on the bedside nurse's appreciation of what a specialist can provide.

Without operative professional responsibility at the bedside, an appreciation of the specialist's practice competence and advocacy of the treatment regimen is less assured. Line authority may be necessary to legitimize authority. The instruments of power may be performance appraisals and rewards for quality car through salary increases and promotion. Different role components will assume prominence depending on staff or line assugnments. Line authority means assuming more direct responsibility for others and presumes the importance of managerial skills.

AN ORGANIZATIONAL MODEL

Clinical specialists have been less than enthusiastic about positions that include line authority. Discontent focuses on an inability to establish clinical work as a priority because of the burden of primary management. The substance of clinical nursing and the heavy demands of 24-hour institutional coordination creates an overwhelming situation in which complex clinical situations tend to be accorded lesser importance. Appreciating this fact, a distinction between administrative and clinical affairs seems justified.

A model of this may be found in the experience of the Rutgers Teaching Nursing Home. The administrative model in this 600-bed nursing home includes a primary administrator, who is responsible for day-to-day operations and delegates authority for the unit, personnel, and patient care management decisions to head nurses; and a clinical chief who delegates authority for the standard of care to clinical directors. The roles of director for clinical affairs, or clinical chief, and clinical director represent the innovation in the model. The clinical directors have been educated as clinical specialists. Each clinical director will eventually be responsible for about 180 beds or three units in the home, with head nurses assigned to a 60-bed unit. The clinical director's job description is currently under development but includes the following broad areas of responsibility:

- Maintaining the standard of clinical care.

- Ensuring that staff have the necessary knowledge and skill to comply with the standards.

- Consulting with staff concerning the management of complex nursing situations.

- Delivering direct care to residents when clinically appropriate.

- Serving as primary caretaker for residents on their units.

This model and its underlying philosophy create new questions. Does clinical policy limit the options in primary management decisions? Figure 1 presents one conceptualization of an organizational chart. To complement the presence of clinically sophisticated nurses in line positions, additional clinical specialists hold staff appointments and serve as tertiary providers. The nature of their specialization reflects the unique needs of the home's case mix. In the Rutgers Teaching Nursing Home, experts in psychogerontology seem most needed. They service the entire home on a referral basis. It is conceivable that such individuals could even be contracted for independently and reimbursed on a fee-for-service basis or shared among several institutions.

Using the clinical specialist in a role as conceived here presents a variety of challenges for nursing education. Clinical preparation must be rigorous and build interdisciplinary collegiality. The best situation would provide for joint education of a variety of professional health care providers. Preparation would also acknowledge that most clinical specialists will work through other people to reach the patient. Skills basic to delegation of responsibility, supervision, and interpersonal effectiveness should be vigorously conveyed.

SUMMARY

The changing health care delivery scene provides nurses a rare opportunity to demonstrate their financial contribution to hospitals. A dramatic contribution can be made by the clinical specialist. To achieve

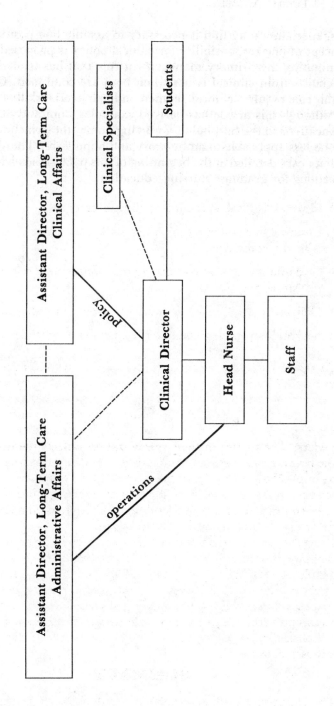

Figure 1. Conceptualization of Organizational Structure for Nursing

Assistant Director, Long-Term Care Administrative Affairs

Assistant Director, Long-Term Care Clinical Affairs

Clinical Specialists

Students

Clinical Director

Head Nurse

Staff

policy

operations

this, specialists may find it necessary to assume line positions. A new concept of line responsibility for clinical policy is proposed, therefore, eliminating the primary management role that has tended to distract specialists from clinical issues when both are combined. Competence in this role requires clinical acumen and managerial skill of high order.

Although this article has derived examples from and demonstrated applications to the hospital and nursing home, the principles discussed are no less applicable to ambulatory and home care. The shift to community care detailed at the beginning of this paper holds additional implications for graduate nursing education.